NOT JUST ABOUT
FOOD

Understanding Eating Disorders

CAROL SONENKLAR WITH TABITHA MORIARTY

TWENTY-FIRST CENTURY BOOKS / MINNEAPOLIS

Twenty-First Century Books™
An imprint of Lerner Publishing Group, Inc.
241 First Avenue North
Minneapolis, MN 55401 USA

For reading levels and more information, look up this title at www.lernerbooks.com.

Diagrams on pages 9, 43, 71 by Laura K. Westlund.
Main body text set in Conduit ITC Std.
Typeface provided by International Typeface Corp.

Library of Congress Cataloging-in-Publication Data

Names: Sonenklar, Carol, author.
Title: Not just about food : understanding eating disorders / Carol Sonenklar.
Description: Minneapolis : Twenty-First Century Books , [2023] | Series: Healthy living library | Includes bibliographical references and index. | Audience: Ages 11–18 | Audience: Grades 10–12 | Summary: "In the United States, approximately 30 million people suffer from an eating disorder. The prevalence of disordered eating among teens and young adults makes this a timely, informative, and helpful book for readers. Learn about the causes, symptoms, and diagnosis of eating disorders as well as treatments. Resources for identifying, treating, and recovering from eating disorders are provided in the text"—Provided by publisher.
Identifiers: LCCN 2021041551 (print) | LCCN 2021041552 (ebook) | ISBN 9781541588943 (library binding) | ISBN 9781728419121 (ebook)
Subjects: LCSH: Eating disorders—United States—Juvenile literature. | Eating disorders—Treatment—Juvenile literature.
Classification: LCC RC552.E18 S593 2023 (print) | LCC RC552.E18 (ebook) | DDC 616.85/2606—dc23/eng/20211013

LC record available at https://lccn.loc.gov/2021041551
LC ebook record available at https://lccn.loc.gov/2021041552

Manufactured in the United States of America
1-47457-48022-4/25/2022

CONTENTS

EATING DISORDERS CAN AFFECT ANYONE

Humans have a complex relationship with eating. It is about much more than basic survival. Certain foods can hold strong associations with our cultures, traditions, families, and memories. One might think of cake and ice cream as birthday party essentials; Seder might call matzah to mind; nian gao may remind someone of Chinese New Year; and black eyed peas and collard greens may be a Kwanzaa favorite. Meals are more than just sustenance for our bodies—they also build our social and emotional connections. Food is often the focus of social gatherings. Many families come together at the dining table to share daily experiences. Friends may meet for coffee or stop at a food truck on the way home from school. These activities strengthen bonds and help us to connect with others.

Western society has propagated a culture that fixates on the weight, shape, and size of the human body. Social media influencers post edited photos depicting impossible beauty standards; video

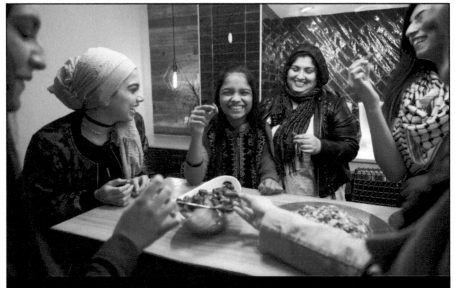

Friends and family often develop traditions around certain foods, such as eating dates to break fast during Ramadan.

streaming services recommend exercise routines that target specific "trouble spots"; and businesses continually market short-term fad diets that contribute to the normalization of an unhealthy relationship with food and body.

Juice "cleanses"; intermittent fasting; and keto, paleo, low-carb, and low-fat diets—among others—have normalized restrictive eating behaviors. It is no wonder that many people experience some sort of disordered eating pattern or unhealthy relationship with food.

While societal ideals and trends can put pressure on individuals to have a certain body weight or shape or to engage with food in a certain way, researchers who study eating disorders are unlikely to point to them as the sole reason a person develops an eating disorder. That's because disordered eating is not just about food or body image. Genetics, physical environment, and psychological and emotional health are all factors in the development of eating disorders.

   While this book will outline some of the most common eating disorders and their symptoms, it is worth noting that each individual is different and may exhibit different symptoms from what are listed. A person may not have all of the symptoms outlined for a particular diagnosis, or they may have symptoms from several different kinds of eating disorders. They could engage in abnormal or unhealthy behaviors that are not mentioned here. No pattern of disordered eating is normal, and there is no "line" between when someone can or should be helped by a professional. If you feel that you or someone you know has disordered eating patterns, even if there is not a clinical diagnosis, you deserve support. Seeing a therapist can be helpful for someone experiencing any sort of disordered or dysmorphic relationship with food or their body.

What Is an Eating Disorder?

The term *eating disorder* can refer to any of a group of psychological disorders characterized by abnormal eating habits. This can include undereating, overeating, bingeing, purging, avoiding certain food groups, and obsessing over exercise. People with eating disorders have an obsession with food and body weight. The way that someone with an eating disorder thinks about food and body weight is very different from the way someone without an eating disorder thinks about the same things. Whereas a person with healthy behaviors may think about food only during mealtimes or when grocery shopping, someone with an eating disorder may spend over 95 percent of their time thinking about food—what they've eaten, how much they ate, and when they will eat again.

A person with an eating disorder may become fraught with anxiety, fear, or panic when thinking about food. They may not want to eat and think of reasons to avoid it. Or they might feel out of control around food and feel they have to punish themselves after eating. Someone with an eating disorder has lost the ability to perceive eating for what it is—a means of staying healthy and alive. Instead, it can be a combative, uncomfortable, or humiliating experience.

In addition to anxiety, individuals dealing with eating disorders often have a distorted perception of how they look. Their disorder prevents them from having a realistic understanding of how they look. Such issues with body image can motivate a person to engage in unhealthy eating behaviors.

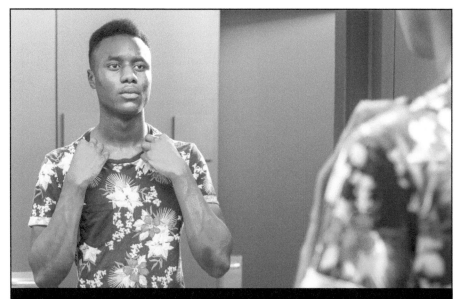

Distorted body image, also called body dysmorphia, can lead to feelings of discomfort, anxiety, and depression. Left untreated, body dysmorphia can significantly interfere with everyday life.

The causes of these disorders are complex. Often eating disorders are triggered by a specific life event, such as a family crisis, an emotional rejection, abuse, or the onset of a psychological disorder. To feel as if they are in control of their lives, people with eating disorders react to these triggers by controlling what they eat.

In the United States, at least 30 million people have an eating disorder. There are many myths about eating disorders, which can discourage people from seeking treatment. Here are a few:

MYTH	FACT
Men do not experience eating disorders.	10 million of the 30 million people who have an eating disorder in the United States are men.
Everyone who has an eating disorder eventually gets help.	An estimated 70 percent of those who have an eating disorder do not receive treatment due to barriers like the stigma around eating disorders or inadequate access to medical care. Many people are embarrassed to admit they have an eating disorder.
Only affluent young white women have eating disorders.	People of all ages and backgrounds have eating disorders. Research shows 13 percent of women over age fifty have symptoms of an eating disorder. Additionally, Black and Hispanic teenagers have higher rates of disordered eating patterns than their white counterparts.
Everyone who has an eating disorder is underweight.	35 percent of people who have binge eating disorder and 30 percent of people who have bulimia are medically obese. Medically overweight and obese people can also experience restrictive eating disorders such as anorexia. You cannot tell that someone has an eating disorder just by looking at them.

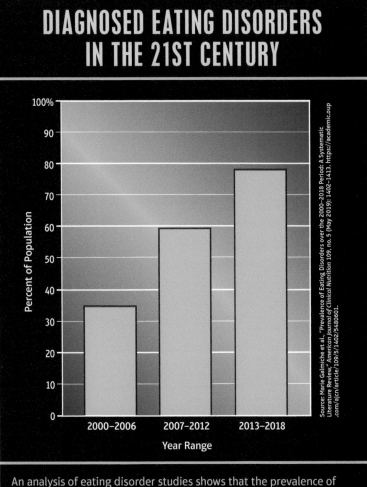

DIAGNOSED EATING DISORDERS IN THE 21ST CENTURY

Percent of Population

Year Range

Source: Marie Galmiche et al., "Prevalence of Eating Disorders over the 2000–2018 Period: A Systematic Literature Review," *American Journal of Clinical Nutrition* 109, no. 5 (May 2019): 1402–1413, https://academic.oup .com/ajcn/article/109/5/1402/5480601.

An analysis of eating disorder studies shows that the prevalence of reported eating disorders has increased over the last two decades, from 3.5 percent to 7.8 percent.

Eating disorders require treatment by a team of professionals. Even with treatment, many people who've engaged in disordered eating work throughout their lives to maintain healthy eating habits and attitudes around food and body image.

A 2019 study showed that the percentage of reported eating disorders is increasing worldwide. Having or knowing a loved one with an eating disorder can be frightening and bewildering. This book will help you understand what causes eating disorders, why they are so difficult to address, and how recovery is possible.

CHAPTER ONE

DISORDERED EATING THROUGH HISTORY

Historical descriptions of people participating in disordered eating behaviors date back to ancient Egypt, Greece, Rome, and Arabia. For example, hieroglyphics from around 1500 BCE show purging was practiced medicinally as a way to prevent foodborne illness.

During the twelfth and thirteenth centuries, Western Christians considered self-starvation a religious act. Women starved themselves to "cleanse their spirits" and become closer to God. One of these women, Saint Catherine of Siena, believed that yielding to hunger was yielding to sin.

In sixteenth-century England, "miraculous maids" claimed to be able to live without nourishment. These women usually came from poor families in rural areas. As news of their miraculous existence spread, people paid to see them. Some of these young women were found to be frauds. Others died of malnutrition.

Historians and doctors debate whether these historical accounts should be included in the history of eating disorders. Some argue that the motivations behind these purging and fasting behaviors—for health and religious purity—are completely different from the drive for thinness that dominates discussions of eating disorders today. Others believe that these are manifestations of disordered eating influenced by sociocultural norms of the day.

Terms for unusual eating behaviors emerged in the English lexicon before there was significant medical research on the subject of eating disorders. Merriam-Webster dates the earliest known use of the word *bulimia* to the fourteenth century, used to mean an abnormal, constant craving for food. Etymologists pinpoint the first use of *anorexia* to 1598, when it meant a prolonged loss of appetite.

Richard Morton, William Gull, and Charles Lasègue

In 1689 an English physician named Richard Morton described a condition that he called *nervous consumption*. The patient he described experienced weight loss and a lack of appetite. The illness was, Morton claimed, caused by "sadness and anxious cares." Most medical historians point to this report as the first modern case of anorexia nervosa. But there would not be any further study of the disorder for another two centuries.

English physician William Gull published the first medical paper on anorexia nervosa in 1873. The report outlined the cases of three emaciated women Gull had treated. Their symptoms included lack of appetite, loss of menstrual period, slow pulse, and slow breathing. The patients' lack of appetite, Gull thought, was caused by an unhealthy mental state rather than a digestive disorder.

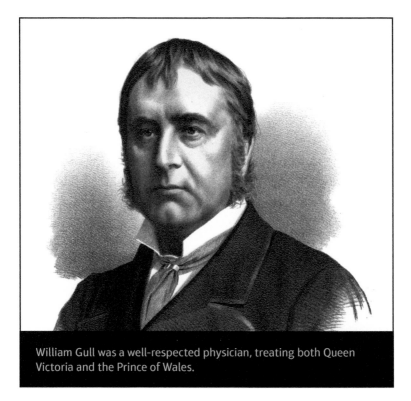

William Gull was a well-respected physician, treating both Queen Victoria and the Prince of Wales.

Charles Lasègue, a French neurologist, published a paper in the same year describing what he called *l'anorexie hystérique* (hysterical anorexia). The symptoms he described aligned with those that Gull had outlined for anorexia nervosa. Gull was excited to find his research substantiated, but he rejected Lasègue's use of the term hysterical, which at the time described emotional problems that affected only women. Gull preferred anorexia nervosa, which referred to a disorder of the central nervous system. To treat anorexia, Gull suggested removing patients from the home. He had observed that anxious parents gave in when the person with anorexia did not want to eat. They would excuse their daughter from eating rather than forcing the issue for fear she would react violently.

HYSTERIA AND WOMEN'S HEALTH

The word *hysteria* comes from the Greek *hysterikos*, which means "a disturbance of the womb." The ancient Greeks believed that the uterus moved around within a woman's body and that certain medical problems were caused by this shifting.

In the 1800s hysteria was a catchall term for a variety of issues and disorders, including fainting, anxiety, and insomnia. A woman could be diagnosed as hysterical for being unhappy, disagreeable, or for going against the wishes of her father or husband, who was typically responsible for making decisions about her clothing, friends, and activities.

Nineteenth-century treatments for hysterical conditions were experimental and often harmful to the patient. Doctors treated women with unproven concoctions that contained lead and mercury. Women could be committed to asylums for a myriad of reasons, including disobeying their male guardians.

Charles Lasègue's interpretation of anorexia as a hysterical condition stems from this misogynistic approach to women's

Hilde Bruch

In 1933 Hilde Bruch immigrated to the United Kingdom because of rising anti-Semitism in her native country of Germany. Bruch was a practicing pediatrician. She began to research childhood obesity in 1937. She then left pediatrics to study psychiatry at Johns Hopkins University in Baltimore, Maryland. She eventually opened a private psychiatric practice and joined the faculty of Columbia University health. In his paper, Lasègue told of an adolescent girl he believed was manipulating her family by refusing to eat. He saw her condition as symbolic of a conflict between maturing daughters and their families. By refusing food, young women could assert power and control without seeming unfeminine. Of course, there is also the possibility that this particular young girl had an eating disorder.

Misguided and sexist treatment of women's mental health issues continued into the twentieth century. Unhappy women or women deemed "uncooperative" were given lobotomies, electroshock therapy, and prescription tranquilizers to pacify them rather than having their emotions taken seriously and being properly treated.

While medical authorities no longer recognize hysteria as a medical disorder, misogyny in women's health continues. In 2022, women continue to be misdiagnosed or have their pain dismissed by doctors as psychosomatic. Those with eating disorders can be dismissed and labeled as attention-seeking rather than receiving the treatment they need.

in New York City. In the 1960s Bruch became interested in anorexia nervosa and began to develop her own theories about the disorder.

Bruch observed that her anorexic patients lacked a sense of self. Bruch discovered through interviews that her patients felt helpless in every part of their lives. Controlling their bodies was an attempt to eliminate the feeling of complete powerlessness.

In 1978 Bruch published *The Golden Cage: The Enigma of Anorexia Nervosa*. In the book, the golden cage represented the middle-class homes of her young patients. She believed they felt trapped. Bruch also found that all her patients with anorexia had distorted perceptions of their appearance and did not recognize how much damage they were doing to their bodies by refusing to eat. Bruch developed a new type of therapy that focused on listening to patients. This approach, called active listening, helped patients with self-esteem issues, which are one of the main contributing factors to developing anorexia. Reported cases of anorexia increased following the publication of Bruch's book.

Doctors didn't know much about anorexia nervosa in the 1970s. Only a few doctors diagnosed and treated it, and those doctors tended to treat patients from upper-class white families. So people assumed that girls from these kinds of families were the only ones

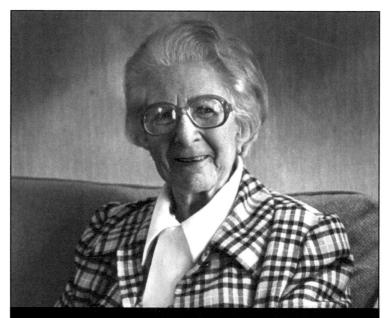

Hilde Bruch was a pioneer in diagnosing and treating anorexia nervosa. She passed away on December 15, 1984.

to have eating disorders. This is untrue—in fact, there are many reasons why people from different backgrounds are unable to seek out treatment for their eating disorders. Systemic barriers to health care and prejudice in the medical field can make it challenging for people of color to reach a diagnosis. Disordered eating behaviors modeled over generations and passed off as "normal" can also delay a person from seeking help.

A Shift in Ideals

After World War II (1939–1945), the Western definition of female beauty shifted. To be beautiful in this new age, a woman had to be thin. Advertisements and other media presented extra weight as disgraceful and indicative of a lack of self-control. Doctors reported that an increasing number of patients were saying they were ashamed of their weight. These people often engaged in disordered eating behaviors such as self-starvation or bingeing and purging.

Gerald Russell

In the 1970s doctors became more aware of patients who gorged themselves on food but maintained a healthy weight. The first description of this behavior as separate from anorexia was by Gerald Russell, a British physician. Russell called bulimia "an ominous variant" of anorexia. He listed three signs that doctors should look for: episodic overeating, laxative misuse, and fear of fatness. Russell believed that female students attending universities were the most likely to have bulimia. Doctors considered bulimia to be a concern only for wealthy families in developed countries.

Growing Awareness

In 1983 Karen Carpenter, one of the most famous singers in the United
States, died of heart failure related to her years-long struggle with
anorexia nervosa. She was only thirty-two. After her death, anorexia
became a topic of considerable media attention, and the public began
to truly understand the seriousness of eating disorders.

HOW COMMON ARE EATING DISORDERS?

According to the National Eating Disorders Association
(NEDA):

- 30 million people in the United States experience
  eating disorders.
- Males represent 25 percent of individuals with
  anorexia nervosa and bulimia nervosa and
  36 percent of individuals with binge eating disorder.
- In a longitudinal study that followed 496 adolescent
  girls for 8 years, 13.2 percent of the girls met
  criteria for an eating disorder by age twenty.
- Binge eating disorder is three times more common
  than anorexia and bulimia combined. Binge eating
  disorder is also more common than breast cancer,
  HIV, and schizophrenia.
- 97 percent of people hospitalized for an eating
  disorder had one or more co-occurring mental
  health conditions.
- The majority of people with eating disorders do not
  receive adequate care.

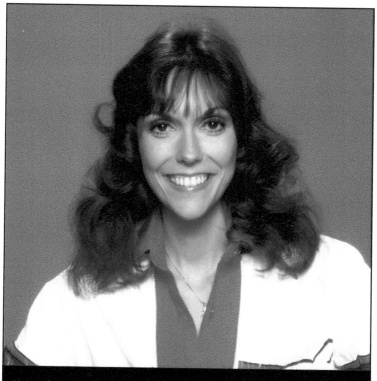

Karen Carpenter is considered one of the greatest vocalists of all time. Her death led to increased visibility and awareness of eating disorders.

Even so, it took many more years for the public to recognize that people of all ethnic and economic backgrounds experienced eating disorders and deserved to get treatment.

More recently, in an effort to help others, several celebrities have spoken out about their battles with eating disorders. Zayn Malik, Taylor Swift, Tyler Oakley, and Camila Mendes are among those who have shared their experiences and sought help.

CHAPTER TWO

TYPES OF EATING DISORDERS

Traditionally anorexia nervosa and bulimia were the only medically diagnosable eating disorders. However, recent research has significantly expanded our understanding of disordered eating. This chapter will examine a few of the most common eating disorders and their common symptoms. However, it's important to remember that disordered eating can manifest in numerous ways. A person may experience only some symptoms or have wide-ranging symptoms beyond what is discussed here. Speaking to a medical professional is the best way to explore one's individual concerns around or symptoms of disordered eating.

Anorexia Nervosa

The word *anorexia* comes from the Greek words *an*, which means "not," and *orexis*, "appetite" or "desire." *Nervosa* means "having to

HOW DOCTORS DIAGNOSE

The descriptions of eating disorders in this book are based on the fifth edition of the *Diagnostic and Statistical Manual of Mental Disorders,* or *DSM-5.* Published by the American Psychiatric Association, the *DSM-5* was written by hundreds of leading experts in the field of psychiatry and mental health and is the manual for officially diagnosing mental health disorders. This edition was published in 2013.

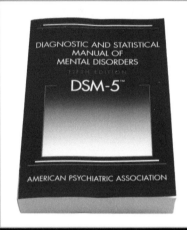

The *DSM-5* updated requirements for diagnosing specific eating disorders and introduced new eating disorder diagnoses that were not included in the previous edition.

do with the nerves." People with anorexia nervosa have an intense fear of gaining weight, to the point where they will severely restrict their caloric intake. This results in an abnormally low body weight. To avoid consuming calories, a person with anorexia may deny hunger, make excuses to avoid eating, or hide food they claim to have eaten. Additionally, they may exercise excessively to burn calories or purge through vomiting or misusing medications such as laxatives or diuretics. A common symptom of anorexia is body dysmorphia—a preoccupation with an imagined or slight physical flaw of one's body. Someone with anorexia may be disturbed by their body weight or the shape of their body. Often they do not recognize when their body is below a healthy weight or the risks of being severely underweight. Although it is an obsession with the physical body, anorexia does not have a purely physical cause. It is a complicated disorder with emotional, psychological, and biological triggers.

There are two main subtypes of anorexia. Some people may only experience one of the types of anorexia, but often a person's disordered eating practices overlap these categories.

Some people with anorexia restrict food altogether, starving themselves. This is known as restrictive type, and it is the type most people are familiar with when talking about anorexia. People with this type allow themselves very few calories each day. They might use diet pills to control appetite or make excuses to avoid eating.

The second type of anorexia is binge/purge type. With this subtype of anorexia, an individual purges food through vomiting, fasting, or misusing laxatives or enemas—a liquid introduced through the anus to stimulate clearing of the bowels. A person with this type of anorexia may also binge, or eat a large amount of food in a short amount of time. The behaviors present in this type of anorexia can be similar to those in bulimia nervosa. However, individuals with this type meet the anorexia criterion of being underweight.

A person with either type of anorexia may control their weight with compulsive exercise. Someone with anorexia will go beyond a healthy amount of exercise. They will exercise under any condition in order to burn calories. They may carry out this excessive exercise in secret, hiding in a bedroom or a bathroom or exercising late at night.

DIAGNOSING ANOREXIA

Anorexia is difficult to diagnose. Many people show only some of the signs of anorexia. Others have symptoms that are not necessarily related to anorexia. Someone with the following symptoms may be in the beginning stages of anorexia:

- a weight that is 15 percent lower than normal for height and age
- an intense fear of becoming fat
- a distorted body image
- symptoms of one type of anorexia: binge/purge type or restrictive type

Atypical anorexia nervosa is just as serious. Atypical anorexia nervosa is when someone meets all of the criteria for anorexia nervosa except for the underweight requirement. This type of anorexia can still cause organ and heart failure.

Anorexia can be a deadly disease. According to the South Carolina Department of Mental Health, 20 percent of people who have anorexia will die prematurely due to complications from their eating disorder, the most common of which are heart failure and suicide.

CHARACTERISTICS OF ANOREXIA

People with anorexia are obsessed with their weight and being thin. Some people may consider the health effects of carrying excess weight and set goals around maintaining a healthy body weight, but anorexia is about more than physical health.

Perfectionism is a common trait for people who develop anorexia. Perfectionists set unrealistically high expectations for themselves and are often highly self-critical. Someone with poor self-image may starve themselves to achieve a "perfect" degree of thinness. They may feel that giving in to their hunger is weak and that if they eat, it proves that they do not have control over their bodies and their lives. Obsession with attaining perfection, combined with a distorted body image, makes it incredibly difficult for someone with anorexia to stop the cycle of dieting and weight loss.

HOW ANOREXIA BEGINS

Anorexia most commonly emerges during adolescence. This is an intensely emotional time. Anorexia is often a physical reaction to things such as stress, anxiety, unhappiness, and a perceived lack of control. The disorder can develop from situations such as doing poorly in school, not being accepted into a group, or failing to make a team or club. People experiencing anorexia often try to establish a sense of control by actively resisting their need to eat.

Adolescence is also a time when your body is changing. As bodies change, it's common for teens to experience body dysmorphia. Especially as sexual characteristics appear and develop, adolescents may become uncomfortable with their body or feel disconnected from it. Some people might find that these physical changes make them want to begin a diet program. Diets can be healthy if there's a positive motivation behind them— say, a desire to increase nutrients by eating more fruits and vegetables, or to reduce or eliminate animal products to cut down

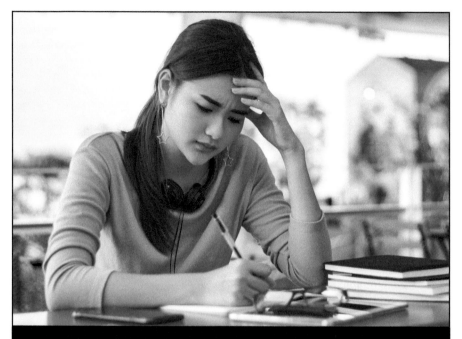

A person experiencing school-related stress or anxiety may turn to disordered eating as a way to cope or feel in control.

on cholesterol or help the environment. But some young people have a completely different relationship with dieting. They may begin to lose weight while dieting and be praised for it. They come to associate their self-worth with being thin. To continue losing weight, they begin to take extreme measures such as fasting, purging, or overexercising. Now this behavior has crossed the line into disordered eating.

"Pressure to diet . . . can be the gateway to anorexia nervosa," affirms Angela Guarda, director of the Eating Disorders Program at John Hopkins University. "Losing those first five to ten pounds, in someone who is genetically vulnerable, seems to make further dieting increasingly compelling and rewarding."

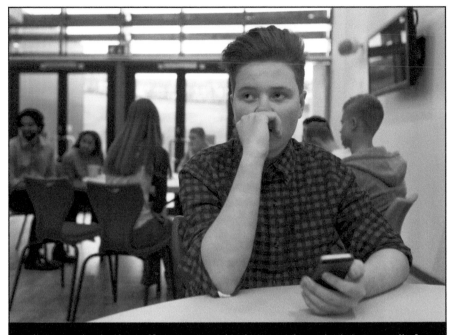

Bullying can lead to low self-esteem, social isolation, and poor body image—all of which can contribute to the development of an eating disorder.

In some cases, a person develops anorexia as a response to a traumatic event. The death of a loved one, parental divorce, sexual assault, a car accident, or a painful breakup may leave a person feeling anxious, depressed, or that their life is out of their control. Bullying, especially in relation to a person's appearance or weight, can negatively impact an individual's body image. They may turn to disordered eating behaviors as a way to avoid dealing with their emotions. These unhealthy coping strategies, if left unchecked, can develop into an eating disorder.

Research suggests that certain individuals are at greater risk of developing anorexia. For example, people who participate in sports that emphasize appearance, such as ballet, wrestling, gymnastics, or bodybuilding, are more likely to develop anorexia than other people. Anorexia is also more common in girls and women than in boys and men, though the number of reported eating disorders in men and boys has increased, possibly in response to growing social pressures around body image, or as seeking help for eating disorders becomes less stigmatized.

Bulimia Nervosa

The word *bulimia* comes from the Greek word *bous*, which means "ox," and the Greek word *limos*, which means "hunger." Bulimia is an eating disorder in which a person binges and then purges. During a binge episode, a person will eat an abnormally large amount of food in a short period of time. It would not be unusual for someone to eat an entire day's worth of calories or more. When someone is bingeing, they almost always binge on junk food or fast food. Someone with bulimia may binge at work, at school, at home, or in restaurants.

Binge episodes tend to be marked by feelings of shame, guilt, or disgust. A person who is bingeing typically knows that they are eating excessively and tries to hide their behavior. Many binges occur at night when everyone else is sleeping. They might sneak food out of their home in the middle of the night to avoid getting caught. They might order large quantities of takeout food and pretend that more people are waiting to eat. Someone on a binge might drive to fast-food restaurants or convenience stores in different towns so the employees do not recognize them. Someone who works in restaurants might take food from people's plates or hide some to take home. Someone on a binge may even take food from a dumpster or trash can.

Bingeing is often accompanied by a feeling of powerlessness. The person might feel as though they're in a trance, or hypnotized. They may ignore any feelings of fullness or discomfort and continue to eat until there is no more food available to eat.

Someone with bulimia will usually purge after the binge, when they feel guilt and remorse over what they have just done. Purging usually takes the form of self-induced vomiting, but people may also turn to laxative misuse, fasting for extremely long periods of time, or excessive exercising as a way to purge the calories they have just consumed. Someone might even purge after any meal or snack, not just after a binge.

If someone is purging by vomiting, it is common to use a finger or an object to touch the back of the throat to stimulate the gag reflex. When done on a daily basis or even more frequently, vomiting becomes easier. Eventually many people with bulimia become able to vomit at will. Someone who engages in vomiting as a form of purging will usually try to hide it. They may run water in the bathroom to cover up the sound, brush their teeth often, or frequently use mints and gum to mask the smell of vomit.

Someone may also turn to laxative misuse to purge after a binge. Laxatives stimulate the digestive system, causing waste products to be eliminated more quickly. Someone misusing laxatives as a method of purging typically believes that this will keep their body from absorbing calories. This is incorrect. Calories from food are absorbed in the small bowel, and laxatives work mainly in the large bowel. The small bowel is very efficient at absorbing calories, no matter how quickly the food moves through the system. Laxatives do not affect the absorption of calories. The only weight a person "loses" with a laxative comes from water.

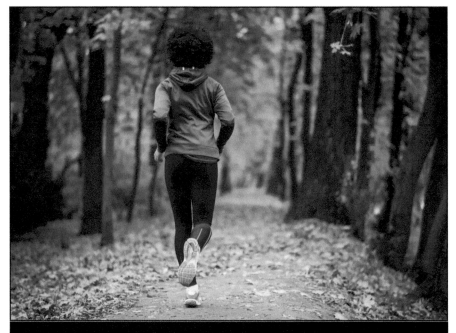

Someone experiencing exercise compulsion may feel distressed if they cannot exercise, or they may exercise despite having a serious injury or illness.

Someone who uses laxatives frequently will eventually develop a tolerance. This means that they need to take a higher dose for the laxative to work. Overusing laxatives this way causes inflammation of the intestinal lining, damage to the colon, and severe dehydration. It can also lead to decreased levels of potassium and sodium, which are important nutrients. Overuse of laxatives can also cause constipation.

Someone trying to purge may also overuse enemas, a liquid that clears the bowel. As with laxatives, enemas can cause dehydration and rectal irritation. Someone with bulimia will often take pains to hide their laxative and enema use. They may clean the toilet bowl rigorously after defecating and spray air freshener.

WARNING SIGNS OF BULIMIA

Because someone with an eating disorder almost always tries to hide it, detecting one is often difficult without an obvious sign such as drastic weight loss. In those with bulimia, it is even harder to notice.

Here's what to look for:

- dieting obsessively
- avoiding a widening range of foods
- avoiding food until certain hours
- anger at others if pressed to eat something
- fear of overeating or gaining weight from a particular meal or type of food
- preoccupation with food, calories, nutrition, and cooking
- not being available for family meals
- denial of hunger
- excessive or compulsive exercising; being overly active
- frequent weighing
- secretive or ritualistic eating
- foods, especially carbohydrates, disappearing quickly from the home
- rapid fluctuations in weight
- depression
- slowness of thought; memory difficulties
- hair loss
- social withdrawal

Some people may take diuretics, which are also known as water pills. Most diuretics are prescription drugs, although some herbal formulas are available. Diuretics draw excess fluid from the body and turn it into urine. As with laxatives, the only weight that is lost comes from water, not from food or calories. Diuretics can be dangerous. They lead to dehydration through excessive urination.

Compulsive exercise is also a type of purging behavior. Someone with bulimia may exercise well beyond what a doctor would consider safe or healthy. Many people struggling with eating disorders will find time and even disrupt other activities to exercise. Like vomiting, they may do it in secret—at night when everyone is sleeping, or in a bathroom, for example. The goal is to "undo" the damage from a binge. People with eating disorders often feel tremendously guilty when they eat anything, not just during a binge. They may exercise excessively to punish themselves and burn the calories.

On the surface, excessive exercise might seem positive. The person may express a desire to get into shape and live a more active lifestyle overall. But this is never the real objective. Exercise, like restricting, bingeing, and purging, gives the person a sense of control over their lives. It is another way to relieve stress and guilt. Overexercising can be addictive. It may become more important than friends, family, school, and just about anything else.

Joint pain, swelling, and stiffness are common in people who overexercise. A person may develop stress fractures in the feet or shins from too-frequent running or hard walking. When combined with food restriction, osteoporosis is a significant risk. Dehydration, loss of the menstrual cycle, and heart and reproductive problems can all result from excessive exercise.

CHARACTERISTICS AND TRIGGERS OF BULIMIA

Bulimia often begins in adolescence or early adulthood, likely for similar reasons as anorexia does. Physiological changes, environmental and emotional stress, and traumatic events may contribute to a person's likelihood of developing bulimia.

As with anorexia, individuals who develop bulimia are preoccupied with their body shape and size and have a fear of gaining weight. Perfectionism is also a common trait of people who develop bulimia. A person with this disorder may judge themselves harshly and have low self-esteem.

Studies have shown that people who participate in bingeing behaviors are more likely to be impulsive, especially if they are feeling stressed. In research conducted by Stanford University, patients were asked to avoid performing a certain task. Those with diagnosed bulimia had significantly more difficulty controlling their impulse to perform the forbidden task. These same patients also had increased brain activity in the frontal lobes, which are responsible for impulse control. Further research may help doctors better understand how to treat patients with bulimia.

Other Recognized Eating Disorders

For a long time, anorexia and bulimia were the only two diagnosable eating disorders. More recently, other types of eating disorders have been recognized by psychologists, medical doctors, and the general public. The *DSM–5* updated diagnostic criteria for anorexia and bulimia and included more types of eating disorders.

Binge eating disorder is the most common eating disorder in the United States, affecting about 1 percent of the general population.

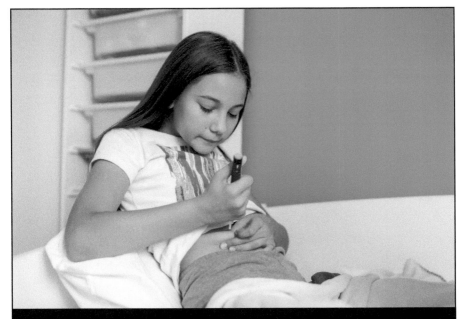

Someone with diabetes needs to pay attention to food, labels, weight, and blood glucose levels in order to stay healthy. This focus on diet and health can put them at increased risk of developing an eating disorder.

A person with binge eating disorder eats large amounts of food in one sitting and has intense feelings of shame or guilt afterward. This binge is usually hidden from friends and family members. Binge eating disorder can manifest similarly to bulimia but with no purging phase.

Diabulimia is an eating disorder that occurs when people with Type 1 diabetes purposefully mismanage their insulin in an attempt to lose weight. This extremely dangerous behavior can quickly become life-threatening. Someone experiencing diabulimia usually exhibits symptoms of other eating disorders as well.

Orthorexia is an obsession with eating foods perceived to be pure, healthy, and nourishing. Someone with orthorexia might avoid

ARFID

In September 2019 many world news organizations circulated the story of a seventeen-year-old in Britain who went blind after a severely restricted diet consisting mainly of potato chips and French fries. His blindness and other physical ailments could have developed from nutritional deficiencies. This individual had ARFID. Someone with ARFID will often exhibit one or more of the following emotions or behaviors:

- severe anxieties related to specific food tastes or textures
- anxiety around vomiting or choking from eating certain foods
- emotional discomfort and disturbance with certain types of foods or textures
- anxiety related to eating around others

entire food groups that they deem unhealthy, feel panicked about food ingredients, and avoid eating completely if a "healthy" food option is not available. Awareness of this disorder has been on the rise recently, with doctors and nutritionists pointing to societal trends as a likely reason.

"Orthorexia is a reflection on a larger scale of the cultural perspective on 'eating cleanly,'" says Sondra Kronberg, founder and executive director of the Eating Disorder Treatment Collaborative. "It centers around eating 'cleanly' and purely, where the other eating disorders center around size and weight and a drive for thinness."

A person may be diagnosed with avoidant/restrictive food intake disorder, or ARFID, if they are extremely selective about the types of food they eat and when they eat them. Some consider this disorder to be an extreme form of "picky eating"; however, this disorder can result in severe nutritional and caloric deficiencies that can require hospitalization. This disorder is very common in children. Often this disorder is not rooted in body image and specific weight loss goals but rather in the textures of food or fears related to food, such as a fear of vomiting or choking.

Other specified feeding or eating disorder (OSFED) is a diagnosis which spans a wide variety of eating disorder symptoms. Someone can experience disordered eating behaviors and thoughts but might not fit into the fairly limiting criteria of other eating disorders like anorexia or bulimia. A diagnosis of OSFED is an important step in getting someone the help they need. OSFED is just as serious as other eating disorders and can be equally detrimental physiologically and psychologically.

CHAPTER THREE

CAUSES OF EATING DISORDERS

E ating disorders are caused by a combination of internal and external forces. Some factors may be biological. Perfectionism, low self-esteem, and other emotional characteristics may also affect whether someone develops an eating disorder. Research suggests that media and other sociological factors could be part of the equation too.

Biological Factors

Until recently, people assumed genetics weren't a factor in developing an eating disorder. But research conducted in 2006 confirmed that eating disorders tend to run in families. A patient is twelve times more likely to develop anorexia and four times more likely to develop bulimia if their mother or sister had it. If one

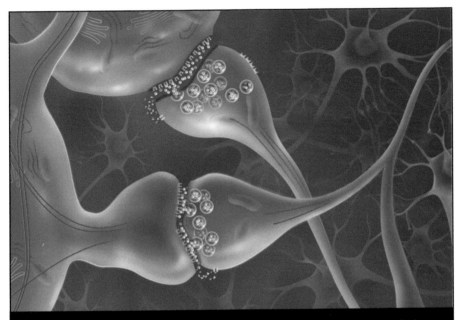

Neurotransmitters (yellow and blue dots) cross the gaps between neurons, called synapses, and are essential to the function of complex neural systems. Scientists have identified more than 500 different types of neurotransmitters in the human body.

identical twin has an eating disorder, their twin has a much greater chance of developing the same disorder.

NEUROTRANSMITTERS

Neurotransmitters transport messages through synapses, the spaces between neurons. These chemicals help control functions such as mood, memory, and appetite. Imbalances in a person's neurotransmitters can cause signals in the brain to misfire.

Serotonin is a type of neurotransmitter that affects many behaviors, including hunger, sleep, impulse control, aggression, anger, depression, anxiety, and perception. If someone has low levels of serotonin, they might be depressed, aggressive, or

COVID-19 AND EATING DISORDERS

In 2019 a new virus that causes severe respiratory illness began to spread around the world. In response to the pandemic, many governments instituted lockdown measures. To prevent the spread of COVID-19, offices, schools, restaurants, and other organizations were required to close. People were encouraged to remain at home. Many employees worked remotely, and educators taught classes through online platforms.

Even before the pandemic, medical experts were concerned about increasing rates of mental illness symptoms, such as depression, in young people. Between 2009 and 2019, the proportion of high school students who reported persistent feelings of sadness and hopelessness increased by 40 percent. The pandemic appears to have exacerbated what was already a concerning situation. A research study covering 80,000 youth worldwide found that depression and anxiety symptoms doubled during the first year of the pandemic. Another study found that over the course of twelve months, there was a 25 percent increase in eating disorder–related

suicidal. High levels of serotonin can lead to anxiety, insomnia, or an obsession with doing everything perfectly. Many doctors believe low serotonin levels may partially explain bingeing behaviors. Consuming sugars and carbohydrates temporarily increases serotonin in the brain and may alleviate symptoms of depression.

hospital admissions compared to prepandemic years for patients between the ages of twelve and eighteen.

Experts believe that the conditions of lockdown created an environment conducive to developing an eating disorder. "The availability of food plays a role," says David Little, one of the authors of the study. "In school you get a lunch break, but you are not surrounded by food. At home, you have access to food all day and night, all the time, healthy or not."

Another explanation may be that fewer eating disorders are going undiagnosed. Being at home also changed family living situations. Parents and caregivers working from home may have been able to identify their child's disordered eating behaviors and helped them receive treatment. A rise in hospitalizations may mean more people were able to get help for their eating disorders.

While children are going back to in-person learning, it's unlikely that the spike in eating disorder cases will go away anytime soon. "It will probably get somewhat better," Little notes, "but until full social structure is back into place, and until . . . we are really back to established routines, this is not going back to baseline."

The neurotransmitter dopamine plays a significant role in how humans experience pleasure. Dopamine production increases when we receive rewards, such as when we get a good grade after studying for a test, or when we eat food that tastes good. Researchers hypothesize that anorexia is related to an overproduction of dopamine. High levels of dopamine increase one's ability to go without pleasurable things such as food. High levels of dopamine may also cause hyperactivity or anxiety. In someone with abnormally high dopamine levels, going without other pleasurable stimuli, which would release more dopamine, can help to manage symptoms such as hyperactivity or anxiety. This is one reason why someone experiencing anorexia may experience relief of anxiety by going without food. Conversely, bulimia has been associated with low dopamine levels, and binge eating is significantly associated with the release of dopamine in the brain.

HORMONES

Hormones are chemicals that control the functions of different tissues and organs. When studying the brains of people with eating disorders, researchers sometimes find that patients have abnormal hormone levels. Doctors are unsure whether such hormone abnormalities contribute to developing an eating disorder or are the effects of one.

Cortisol, a hormone that controls stress and anxiety, is sometimes at high levels in the brains of people with eating disorders. Leptin, a hormone that controls appetite and weight, is sometimes low. Leptin is produced by the body's fat tissue and then released into the bloodstream. In people with very little or no body fat, leptin levels drop. A significant drop in an individual's body fat can affect thyroid function and put them at risk for osteoporosis, a disease that thins and weakens bones.

It is important to remember that biological factors alone do not lead to eating disorders. Many people with irregular neurotransmitter or hormone levels do not develop eating disorders. A combination of internal biological and psychological factors and external environmental factors triggers disordered eating behavior.

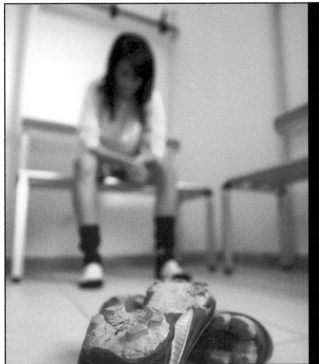

Athletes with perfectionism demand a high quality of performance in both practice and competition. They may feel extremely disappointed when they do not meet their high standards.

Psychological Factors

People with eating disorders tend to share certain psychological traits. Perfectionism, low self-esteem, and judgmental attitudes have all been linked to eating disorders.

People with eating disorders are often very critical of themselves and others. They may perceive the world as black and white, with rarely any middle ground. Someone with an eating disorder may also have low self-esteem. They may feel they will only have value if they lose weight or reach their goal weight. They often feel as though food is the one thing they can control, whether by refusing it or bingeing.

CO-OCCURRING CONDITIONS

Someone who is struggling with an eating disorder is often struggling with other mental illnesses as well. A study of individuals hospitalized for an eating disorder found that 97 percent of them were also struggling with another co-occurring disorder. In this same study, 22 percent of these individuals were struggling with post-traumatic stress disorder (PTSD), 20 percent were struggling with obsessive-compulsive disorder (OCD), and 22 percent struggled with an alcohol or substance use disorder. A similar study found that two-thirds of people with anorexia began experiencing symptoms of anxiety a few years before developing their eating disorder. 73.8 percent of people struggling with binge eating disorder have at least one other major psychiatric diagnosis, and 38 percent of people struggling with OSFED exhibit another disorder as well.

Experiencing a co-occurring disorder can make seeking treatment even more difficult. For example, someone struggling with an eating disorder as well as major depressive disorder might lack the motivation to seek help or change their behavior patterns. Someone struggling with OCD as well as an eating disorder might experience severe anxiety at the thought of changing their current rituals and schedules. It is important that people who are struggling with multiple diagnoses get help and support for each individual diagnosis in order to fully heal and recover.

Some celebrities who have gone public with their struggles with co-occurring disorders include:

- Demi Lovato (bulimia, substance use disorder, bipolar disorder)
- Russell Brand (bulimia and bipolar disorder)

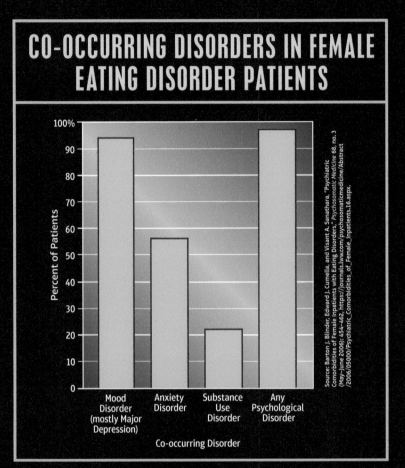

CO-OCCURRING DISORDERS IN FEMALE EATING DISORDER PATIENTS

Percent of Patients

100%, 90, 80, 70, 60, 50, 40, 30, 20, 10, 0

Mood Disorder (mostly Major Depression) | Anxiety Disorder | Substance Use Disorder | Any Psychological Disorder

Co-occurring Disorder

Source: Barton J, Blinder, Edward J. Cumella, and Visant A. Sanathara, "Psychiatric Comorbidities of Female Inpatients with Eating Disorders, *Psychosomatic Medicine* 68, no. 3 (May–June 2006): 454–462, https://journals.lww.com/psychosomaticmedicine/Abstract /2006/05000/Psychiatric_Comorbidities_of_Female_Inpatients.16.aspx.

A 2006 study analyzed hospitalized female eating disorder patients to understand how common it was for someone with an eating disorder to have one of twenty-seven possible co-occurring disorders. The study found that 97 percent of individuals had at least one co-occurring diagnosis, with mood disorders, anxiety disorders, and substance use disorder being the most common.

- Lady Gaga (bulimia, anorexia, depression, PTSD)
- Elton John (bulimia, substance use disorder)
- Stephanie Covington Armstrong, author of *Not All Black Girls Know How to Eat* (bulimia, depression)
- Gabourey Sidibe (bulimia, depression)

43

Perfectionism is strongly associated with eating disorders. Perfectionists believe that they are valued and measured by their achievements—in school, sports, or social circles. As a result, the person's self-esteem is dependent on other people's approval. Perfectionism puts tremendous pressure on a person to excel in all aspects of life.

Perfectionists may feel inferior because they have to work hard to meet the high standards they have set for themselves. These

BODY POSITIVITY AND BODY NEUTRALITY

In recent years, many brands have begun body positivity movements that try to encourage realistic and healthy body expectations. For example, the young women's lingerie brand Aerie launched a campaign in 2014 called "#AerieREAL." With this campaign, Aerie no longer airbrushes their models and tries to use models of all heights, weights, body types, races, and abilities in their marketing ads. Several other brands have begun to follow suit. Models like Katie Willcox and Iskra Lawrence use their social media platforms to spread body positivity and healthy lifestyle habits.

Initially, the body positivity movement provided relief and confidence for many girls and women who began to see bodies that looked like theirs positively represented in advertising and on social media platforms. However, critics of the body positivity movement say that it is unrealistic to feel positively about one's body at all times.

Enter the concept of body neutrality. Body neutrality is the idea that you are not always going to feel good about feelings may result in a distorted self-image and lower self-esteem. This might make perfectionists more vulnerable to developing an eating disorder.

Sociological Factors

Many people blame the increasing number of reported eating disorders on societal influences, particularly mass media. Media

your body every day, and that's OK. Rather than fight to be positive every day, this movement adopts the idea of being neutral about your body. A person with body neutrality appreciates what their body can do while accepting its appearance and limitations. Being body neutral involves not allowing appearance or weight to dictate one's mental state or sense of worth.

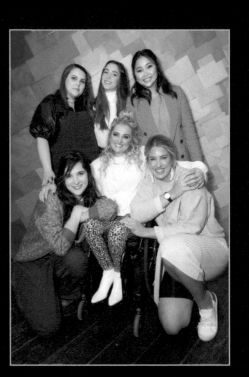

In 2020 Aerie partnered with celebrities, including (*top row, from left to right*) Beanie Feldstein, Aly Raisman, and Lana Condor, to promote their #AerieREAL campaign.

in Europe and North America tends to promote thinness as the ultimate in physical beauty for women. Men are presented with images of large, muscular models with little body fat. Beauty magazines, advertisements, social media posts, and other forms of media achieve these masculine and feminine ideals using photo-editing software. Although the media does not cause eating disorders, exposure to these images can lead people to associate their weight with their self-worth.

In the late 1990s and early 2000s online groups known as "pro-ana" (pro-anorexia) and "pro-mia" (pro-bulimia) platforms were very popular. These groups consisted of people with anorexia and bulimia supporting and egging on one another's disordered behaviors. They did not believe that their conditions were unhealthy; they viewed anorexic and bulimic behaviors as lifestyle choices. These groups were very dangerous, especially because many people in the groups truly believed they were helping one

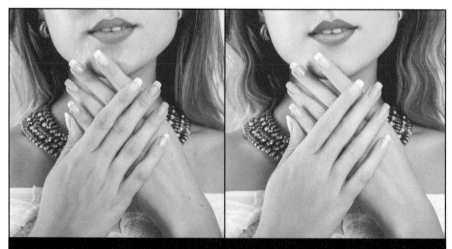

Many businesses use photo-editing software to airbrush models' features to achieve a "perfect" appearance.

another. These groups have now been banned on most popular social media sites. Platforms like Instagram, Facebook, and Tumblr have begun blocking posts and groups that promote unhealthy levels of thinness or are pro-eating disorder. However, while many of these groups are officially banned, communities that promote eating disorders still exist and will likely continue to exist as long as we live in a society that gravitates toward viewing beauty as a physical checklist. These communities may masquerade as promoting health or beauty, but they are still encouraging their followers to engage in harmful practices as a method of achieving so-called health or beauty.

CHAPTER FOUR

WHO GETS EATING DISORDERS?

For a long time, doctors thought that eating disorders affected only affluent, young, white women. But this is no longer the case. In the last twenty years researchers have made leaps and bounds in their understanding of disordered eating. Now doctors recognize that eating disorders can affect anyone, regardless of gender identity, race, age, and socioeconomic status.

Men and Eating Disorders

The first national study of eating disorders was conducted in 2007 by Harvard University researchers. They found that 25 percent of all people with anorexia and 40 percent of all people with bulimia were boys or men. Earlier estimates had put the number of men with eating disorders at just 10 percent.

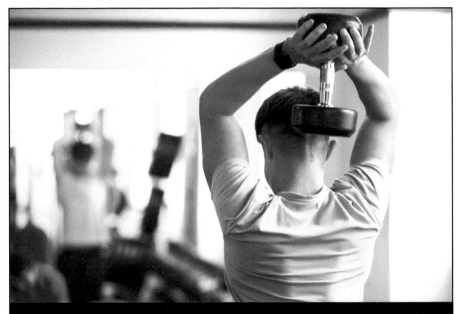

Because exercise is generally considered a positive activity that improves wellness, it can be tough for someone to recognize when exercise becomes problematic.

Boys typically begin disordered eating behavior between the ages of twelve and fourteen, but boys as young as eight years old have been diagnosed. The emotional force behind an eating disorder is usually the same for all genders. A boy might think he has to reshape his body or lose weight to excel at a sport. He might believe that his success as an athlete is what gives him value. He might be teased at home or school for being out of shape or overweight. Making the conscious choice to limit what he eats gives him a sense of power over his life.

The disorder is often triggered by an obsession with fitness and getting in shape. For example, a boy may feel pressure to make a team or be a better player. He starts to eat less and less while increasing his exercise. This may seem at first like a healthy lifestyle choice but can progress to a dangerous situation if left unchecked.

Boys and men are less likely to be diagnosed with an eating disorder due to cultural differences and gender norms. It may take their friends and family longer to recognize that they have an eating disorder. This means a longer time before they can start treatment.

SHAPE VERSUS THINNESS

Boys and men often have a different objective when they want to change their bodies. Young boys may watch shows and movies featuring action heroes with unrealistic body proportions that are impossible to attain. Thin, hard-bodied male models with highly defined, sculpted muscles and six-pack abs grace the covers of men's magazines. Those same photos are billboard-sized in retail stores. Popular baseball and basketball players sometimes take performance-enhancing drugs to increase their strength and muscularity.

Studies have shown that many men and boys who watch commercials with muscular actors become unhappy with their own bodies. Representations of masculinity in the US have been linked to eating disorders and misuse of performance-enhancing drugs.

DIAGNOSIS AND TREATMENT ISSUES

Eating disorders are difficult to diagnose in males. Cultural norms make it difficult for people who identify as male to express body image issues. Boys who are struggling with these problems usually feel intense shame and embarrassment. This makes it difficult for them to admit they have a problem, even with obvious symptoms such as extreme weight loss, bingeing, and purging.

Current standards that doctors use to diagnose eating disorders are based on a very narrow view of who experiences eating disorders and how symptoms can manifest. For example, one of the clinical

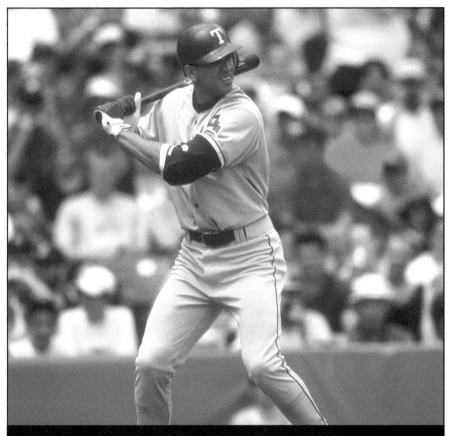

Alex Rodriguez, one of modern baseball's most famous sluggers, admitted to using performance-enhancing drugs while playing for the Texas Rangers from 2001–2003. He said that he felt "an enormous amount of pressure" to succeed, and that the culture in Major League Baseball at the time encouraged the use of performance-enhancing drugs.

signs of anorexia has classically been amenorrhea, or loss of the menstrual cycle. Recent studies have shown that people who experience a menstrual cycle may have a severe eating disorder and still get their period. At the same time, people who do not normally experience menstrual cycles may still have severe eating disorders.

William Rhys Jones, a doctor and member of the Royal College of Psychiatrists in London, England, has emphasized that a lack of understanding and sometimes sympathy for men and boys with eating disorders remain barriers to treatment. "We must continue to address the ongoing gender bias around eating disorders so every man who is suffering feels comfortable to get help when they need it," he said.

Attitudes have slowly begun to change since the publication of the 2007 Harvard study on males and eating disorders. Treatment centers have started specific programs designed for boys and men. Males-only recovery groups allow for open discussion of emotional issues. As a result of a growing awareness of the problem among males, a few celebrities have admitted to their problems. Actors Dennis Quaid and Billy Bob Thornton have both talked about their battles with anorexia and bulimia.

Athletes and Eating Disorders

Studies show that people who compete at high levels of certain performance sports, such as diving and figure skating, are at higher risk for abnormal food behaviors. Athletes at risk for eating disorders include those who feel the pressure of "making weight" to compete, as in wrestling. Coaches often encourage unhealthy eating and exercise habits. Sometimes athletes abuse their bodies for the short-term goals of the team. Ironically, these practices can undermine health and athletic performance in the long run. Although gymnastics and wrestling will be discussed due to their emphasis on body weight, eating disorders in athletes are not restricted to these sports. One study found that one third of Division I female athletes exhibited behaviors that would place them at risk for developing anorexia nervosa. Another study found that 35 percent of female collegiate athletes and 10 percent of male collegiate athletes were at risk for anorexia. This same study found that 58 percent of female and 38 percent of male collegiate athletes were at risk for bulimia nervosa. Increased awareness of what disordered eating behaviors look like and an emphasis on high quality nutrition for performance, promoted by coaches and other adult figures in these athletes' lives, can help combat disordered eating in athletes.

GYMNASTICS

Historically, significant focus has been placed on small body size and low body weight at the elite level of gymnastics. The standard height and weight for gymnasts has changed dramatically over the years. In 1976 the six women on the US Olympic artistic gymnastics team averaged 5 feet 3 inches (160 cm) and weighed 106 pounds (48 kg). In 1992 the average female gymnast was 4 feet 9 inches (145 cm) and weighed 83 pounds (38 kg). Female gymnasts are particularly prone to disordered eating. One in ten male gymnasts also has an eating disorder.

Several famous gymnasts have gone public with their eating disorder experiences. Olympic gymnast Cathy Rigby had bulimia and anorexia for twelve years. She went into cardiac arrest twice because of her anorexia. Rigby recalls that although not as much was known about nutrition when she competed, the coaches told the girls what their weight should be. Rigby weighed about 94 pounds (43 kg) during her Olympic run. She was eating one meal a day to drop her weight to 90 pounds (41 kg), which the coaches set as the mandatory weight. Like many other gymnasts, Rigby had no trouble maintaining that weight until her body started to go through puberty.

53

RED-S

RED-S, or relative energy deficiency in sport, is a syndrome that has been recognized in the medical field in recent years. Formerly called the "female-athlete triad," referring to the common effects of osteopenia (low bone density), amenorrhea (loss of menstrual cycle) and disordered eating in female athletes, the syndrome has now been expanded and adapted to recognize the harmful effects of improper energy intake in all athletes. Relative energy deficiency in sport occurs when a person's food intake is not high enough to maintain their energy output during exercise. While RED-S is not an eating disorder on its own, the effects of RED-S are the effects of undereating, and disordered eating patterns can be a part of the diagnosis of RED-S.

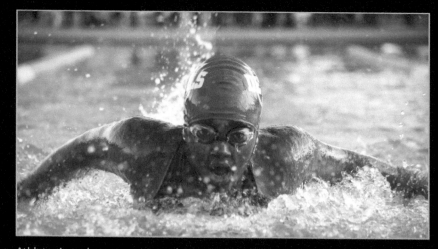

Athletes in endurance sports such as cross-country running, aesthetic sports such as gymnastics, or sports with formfitting uniforms such as swimming, may be at higher risk of RED-S than athletes in other sports.

PHYSICAL/MEDICAL SIGNS AND SYMPTOMS OF RED-S

- dehydration
- gastrointestinal problems
- cold intolerance
- cardiac abnormalities such as low heart rate and low blood pressure
- stress fractures and overuse injuries
- significant weight loss
- muscle cramps, weakness, or fatigue
- dental and gum problems

PSYCHOLOGICAL/BEHAVIORAL SIGNS AND SYMPTOMS

- anxiety or depression
- exercising beyond what's expected or required
- excessive use of the restroom
- lack of focus or difficulty concentrating
- preoccupation with weight and eating
- avoidance of eating and eating situations
- misuse of laxatives, diet pills, or diuretics

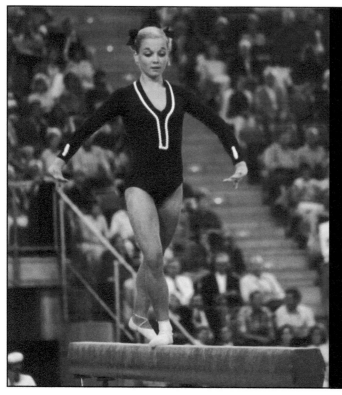

In an interview, Cathy Rigby said she was "obsessed with being the perfect team member," and that she was willing to do anything to meet the goal weight set by her coaches.

Before puberty, girls and boys have similar amounts of body fat, about 16 to 18 percent. When girls begin puberty, their hips widen and they gain more body fat. After puberty, many athletic females try to maintain a low body fat percentage, but it is difficult.

Competing in gymnastics is extremely demanding. Certain psychological traits such as perfectionism, compulsiveness, and high personal expectations are common in gymnasts because these traits can help the athletes succeed in their sport. However, these are also key traits associated with eating disorders.

In recent years, the trends of height and body weight have begun to increase again as gymnastics has moved toward valuing power and strength in performance. In the 2016 Olympics in Rio de Janeiro, Brazil, the US women's gymnastic team had an average height of 5 feet (152 cm) and an average weight of 108 pounds (49 kg). Increased awareness of eating disorders in gymnastics and a push to address them has also majorly influenced this trend.

WRESTLING

Wrestlers are known for their extreme weight-cutting practices to develop the slim, lean build that the sport demands. Cutting to a lower weight class is thought to give a wrestler an advantage against a smaller opponent. Before weighing in for a match, wrestlers may restrict fluids and calories by fasting, purging, using laxatives, and overexercising. These drastic measures allow wrestlers to lose enough weight to drop into a lower class in a short amount of time. Wrestlers have reported doing this as often as ten times a season. Participating in this practice can lead to long-term habits and eventually to an eating disorder.

Eating Disorders and Marginalized Populations

The notion that only heterosexual, young, thin, white females experience eating disorders can be a barrier to other people receiving treatment. This misconception is rooted in the fact that in the 1800s, when eating disorders were first beginning to be recognized and diagnosed by the medical field, those who had access to medical care were affluent white families. Since eating disorders often begin in adolescence, doctors and society developed a bias that eating disorders primarily affect young white females.

ATHLETES AND EATING DISORDERS: WHAT COACHES, PARENTS, AND TEAMMATES NEED TO KNOW

The NEDA created guidelines to increase awareness of warning signs for eating disorders and strategies to help young people avoid developing them.

RISK FACTORS FOR ATHLETES

- sports that focus on appearance or weight requirements, such as gymnastics, diving, and wrestling, or that focus on the individual rather than a team
- endurance sports
- belief that lower body weight will have a positive impact on performance
- early childhood involvement in a sport

As research into eating disorders has progressed and social movements have begun to bring more awareness to the way eating disorders affect people from all backgrounds, the discussion around eating disorders has become more inclusive.

EATING DISORDERS AND PEOPLE OF COLOR

A study conducted in 2009 found that Black teenagers are 50 percent more likely than white teenagers to engage in disordered eating behaviors like bingeing and purging. Hispanic adolescents

- low self-esteem, family problems, family history of eating disorders, chronic dieting, traumatic life experiences
- coaches who focus on success rather than on the athlete as a whole person

HOW TO PROTECT ATHLETES AGAINST EATING DISORDERS

- use a positive coaching style
- ensure the support of teammates with healthy body attitudes
- emphasize using participation in sports as a path to personal success, using motivation and enthusiasm rather than focusing on body weight or shape
- remember that sports should be fun

are also more likely to have bulimia nervosa than non-Hispanic adolescents are. Finally, people of color with self-acknowledged disordered eating behaviors are significantly less likely to have their doctor ask them about those behaviors and are less likely to receive help for eating disorders than their white counterparts are.

Before the 2009 study, doctors thought that cases of eating disorders were rare in people of color. This gap in knowledge might be due to a number of factors. Racial bias in health care may be one reason there is less visibility for people of color with eating disorders. In a 2006 study, when physicians were given identical case studies that presented disordered eating behaviors but gave a different racial background, the physicians were far less likely to identify the behaviors of Hispanic and Black women as problematic than in case studies where the patients were white women. They were also far less likely to recommend that Black women seek help in addressing disordered eating behaviors.

Systemic inequalities in health care can also mean that fewer people of color seek help for eating disorders. People of color have faced longstanding disparities in health insurance coverage compared to coverage for white citizens. While these disparities have shrunk in recent years, people of color are still more likely to be uninsured than their white counterparts. People without insurance do not usually go for regular checkups or seek medical advice except in emergencies.

Beyond the systemic challenges present in health care, some individuals may not feel they can seek help due to cultural norms. In her book *Not All Black Girls Know How to Eat*, Stephanie Covington Armstrong discusses her experience as a woman of color struggling with an eating disorder. "I had an extremely difficult time seeking help because all my life I had been told I needed to fit into the strong Black woman archetype. I felt like a failure and had a lot of shame because of my bulimia and anorexia," she explains. "Although eating disorders are a huge problem in the Black community, we are taught that we must deal with our problems ourselves. Until it becomes socially acceptable for minority women to seek mental health support, they will continue to be isolated in both their community and their disease. We need to go into these areas and educate people on eating disorders and help them to see that seeking help is a sign of strength and not weakness."

EATING DISORDERS IN THE LGBTQIA+ COMMUNITY

According to a 2009 study, men who identify as gay, bisexual, or mostly heterosexual—that is, primarily but not exclusively attracted to the opposite gender—were seven times more likely to report bingeing and twelve times more likely to report purging than straight men were. The same study found that women who identify as lesbian, bisexual, or mostly heterosexual are twice as likely to report binge eating as their heterosexual counterparts are. People in the LGBTQIA+ community face unique stressors and challenges that can contribute to the development of an eating disorder. Some of these may include fear of judgment or rejection by friends and

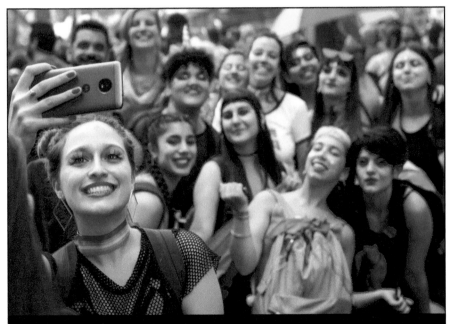

Every June in the United States, members of the LGBTQIA+ community and their allies come together to recognize the impact LGBTQIA+ individuals have had on local, national, and international history. Many cities host Pride marches and events and provide educational resources and services for LGBTQIA+ individuals.

family; unsupportive or dangerous living, working, or learning environments; or dissonance between someone's gender identity and the gender they were assigned at birth.

People in the LGBTQIA+ community can experience additional barriers to getting treatment for an eating disorder. They may live in an area without care that can address the unique gender and sexuality issues that people in the LGBTQIA+ community face. They may lack social support from family and friends who could encourage them to seek help.

However, research has shown that feeling connected in the LGBTQIA+ community is a protective factor against eating disorders. More and more community and health care centers are dedicated to helping members of the LGBTQIA+ community manage all mental health disorders, including eating disorders.

EATING DISORDERS IN OLDER POPULATIONS

Eating disorders can occur at any time of life. Midlife triggers such as pregnancy, divorce, unemployment, or even natural signs of aging can contribute to developing an eating disorder. Additionally, people who have struggled with eating disorders in the past can experience relapses during stressful times. Shame and uncertainty can be major barriers for older populations to seek treatment. They may feel as if they have developed a "teenager's problem." This is untrue. Eating disorders can affect anyone, regardless of age. It is important for people of any age to get help.

YOUNG CHILDREN AND DISORDERED EATING

Adolescence is the most common time for eating disorders to begin. But children as young as five and six years old may be concerned about weight and body image.

Gene Beresin, a Harvard psychiatrist, believes that the onset of anorexia has two peaks: one between the ages of ten and thirteen and the other between the ages of thirteen and eighteen. His research has shown that the majority of younger children who are overly concerned about their weight have mothers who are worried about their own bodies. Mothers who devote a great deal of time and energy to staying slim can strongly influence their children.

According to recent studies, many fifth- and sixth-grade girls have tried to lose weight. This doesn't mean they will develop eating disorders, but it may signal a discomfort with their physical appearance, often connected to the onset of puberty and the accompanying bodily changes such as weight gain, hip widening, and the development of breasts. Disordered eating behaviors can cause serious health problems in everyone, but especially in young, growing children. Nutrient deficiencies caused by disordered eating can do permanent damage to their bodies and leave them with chronic health issues.

EATING DISORDERS AND PEOPLE WITH DISABILITIES

While there is ample independent research about eating disorders and about disability, few studies address the presence of eating disorders in people with disabilities. Some research has shown that people with physical disabilities may be more vulnerable to body dissatisfaction or may be extra sensitive about their body's size and shape. About one-third of people with an intellectual disability have eating or feeding issues that may affect eating behavior. Further research on how disability, body image, and eating disorders overlap is needed to improve diagnosis and treatment options.

People living with a disability and an eating disorder may encounter barriers to getting the help they need. For example, physicians may not ask questions to investigate the presence of disordered eating behaviors because the person's disability masks the effects of the disordered eating. Additionally, many types of treatment programs are not equipped to accommodate someone who is disabled.

FAT PEOPLE AND EATING DISORDERS

The idea that someone must be below a certain weight or body fat percentage to experience an eating disorder is a myth. People of all weights and sizes can have an eating disorder, and they can still experience the incredibly dangerous and harmful effects of malnutrition. Eating disorders often go unrecognized by medical professionals when the person with the disorder is clinically overweight or obese. In fact, they may be praised by their physician, friends, and family for pursuing so-called healthy behaviors. In such cases, a person may never get the help they need, or they may get it only when their disorder has done irreparable damage to their body. Better education and recognition of the effects of malnutrition in people of all weights and sizes can help combat this false belief and remove barriers for fat people to receive help for their eating disorders.

Eating disorders affect all groups of people, and all people deserve to get better. By promoting awareness of the prevalence of eating disorders in all communities, dispelling myths about who develops eating disorders, and redefining what health looks like, we can ensure that people are able to get the help that they need.

CHAPTER FIVE

HOW EATING DISORDERS AFFECT THE BODY

Someone following a severely restrictive eating pattern usually decreases the amount of carbohydrates, fat, and protein in their diet. They eat very low-calorie foods which have little nutritional value. Taking vitamins cannot make up for these losses. Malnutrition affects every organ and system of the body, especially the brain, heart, kidneys, bones, skin, hair, and intestines. Over time, this type of diet leads to a decrease of muscle, called muscle wasting. A person's stomach can swell because of protein deficiency. The effects of malnutrition are serious and can put a person at high risk of injury or death.

Body Fat

Fat is one of the basic components of the body. It is essential for keeping the body functional and healthy. Fat provides padding to

BODY WEIGHT BREAKDOWN

Doctors separate body weight into three types: bone, muscle, and fat. In a typical woman of average weight, bones make up approximately 12 percent of total body weight, muscle and lean tissue about 35 percent, and body fat about 25 percent. In a typical man, bones make up about 15 percent of total body weight, body fat about 10 to 20 percent, and muscle and lean tissue about 40 percent. The remaining body weight comes from skin, connective tissue, tendons, blood, and organs.

protect our organs from damage and insulates our bodies from cold. It is where we store vitamins A, D, E, and K and is the body's main source of energy. Fat cells also play a role in regulating our metabolism and in supporting our immune system.

Restrictive eating disorders often deplete the body's essential fat stores, causing certain biological processes to break down. Without fat, the body cannot absorb certain vitamins, increasing the risk of vision impairment, infertility, loose teeth, swollen gums, and easy bruising, among other issues.

Some body fat lies directly under the skin layers. This is called subcutaneous fat. It contains blood vessels, which supply oxygen to the skin. When subcutaneous fat is lost, the veins in the skin and outline of bones stand out. The body takes on a gaunt, skeletal appearance. Lack of subcutaneous fat in the face may give someone with an eating disorder sunken eye sockets, making the eyes appear to bulge. The scalp will also appear bony and dry.

Metabolism, Glucose, and Hormones

Metabolism is the conversion of food, fluids, and other substances into glucose. Glucose is the body's fuel. Without it, we cannot survive in good health. Restrictive eating disorders limit the amount of food, and therefore glucose, entering the body. In response, a person's metabolism may slow down to conserve energy.

A person with a slowed metabolism may not be able to produce a healthy amount of hormones. Hormones are chemicals that bring information to and from cells. Hormones control nearly all bodily processes. They are involved in bone development, growth, mood regulation, and energy levels. This metabolic slowdown and resulting hormone deficiencies cause issues with numerous body processes.

Someone who doesn't consume enough calories to maintain proper bodily function will often have an abnormally low body temperature, frequently feeling cold even in warm climates. Studies show that people with eating disorders often have gastrointestinal issues such as irritable bowel syndrome (IBS) and heartburn. For those who have not completed puberty, hormone disruption can delay or disrupt sexual development and permanently stunt growth. Amenorrhea is also common.

Electrolytes

Electrolytes, such as calcium and potassium, are essential minerals in the body. They help cells function normally by maintaining an electrical charge across cell membranes. They regulate nerve and muscle function. Restrictive and purging behaviors can lead to dehydration and an electrolyte imbalance. Common symptoms of electrolyte imbalances include headaches, confusion, dizziness,

AMENORRHEA

Amenorrhea is one of the most common symptoms of restrictive eating disorders for people who menstruate. Traditionally, it was even a criterion for diagnosing anorexia. However, numerous conditions can contribute to amenorrhea that are not related to disordered eating.

Emotions and mental health also affect hormones, so excessive stress or pressure can cause amenorrhea. Athletes who train rigorously, such as long-distance runners, gymnasts, or ballet dancers, often lose their periods due to low body fat, stress, and high-energy expenditure. People who use hormonal contraceptives, such as birth control pills or an IUD, may not have periods. Often amenorrhea results from a combination of several of these factors.

nausea, fatigue, and muscle spasms. In severe cases, a person can experience seizures or fall into a coma.

Heart

Heart disease is the number one cause of death for people with anorexia and bulimia. It is a significant concern for other eating disorders as well. Decreased metabolism and an imbalance of electrolytes affect heartbeat and blood pressure. The heart rate of a person with an eating disorder might drop to fewer than sixty beats per minute. They may develop an irregular heartbeat or have chest pains. The strength of their heartbeat may also be weaker, resulting in low blood pressure. This condition can cause headaches, dizziness, and weakness, and severely low blood pressure can deprive the body of enough oxygen to carry out its functions. Someone with an eating disorder might often feel faint or lightheaded, especially when they stand up after lying down. Their hands and feet might also have a bluish tinge due to poor circulation.

Osteoporosis

Bones are living tissues. The body constantly breaks down old bone and builds up new bone. A healthy diet and exercise make bones stronger. When old bone breaks down faster than new bone is made, bone loss occurs. Poor nutrition and decreased body fat can lead to bone loss. Over time, this can cause osteoporosis, a bone disease in which bones break easily and heal slowly. Osteoporosis is a common and dangerous effect of eating disorders.

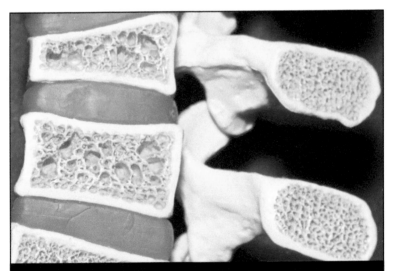

Osteoporosis in the spine can leave vertebrae susceptible to painful fracturing or complete collapse.

Researchers have found that adolescents who have anorexia lose more bone density (solidness of bone) than adults with anorexia do. When bone density decreases, there is a much higher risk of fracturing or breaking a bone. A person with an eating disorder can fracture a bone from any high-impact activity, such as running on hard pavement, or playing a contact sport, such as football, soccer, or basketball.

As we age, our bones weaken, so if individuals lose bone strength in adolescence, they will have problems with weak bones long into adulthood.

Skin and Hair

When confronted with a severe calorie deficit, the body attempts to maintain its most essential organ functions. But to do this, it withholds nourishment from less essential areas. A person with an eating disorder may have brittle nails and dry skin due to lack of protein and fat. Substantial hair loss is also common.

With extreme weight loss, the body no longer has fat to serve as natural insulation. To retain body heat, someone with an eating disorder will often develop downy body hair called lanugo that grows on the back, arms, legs, face, and neck. This type of hair takes fewer calories to produce than normal hair does.

Brain Function

Without energy, the brain cannot function properly. A lack of glucose can cause the brain to slow down and shrink. Low glucose levels can lead to difficulties with both short- and long-term memory. The risks of seizure and stroke increase.

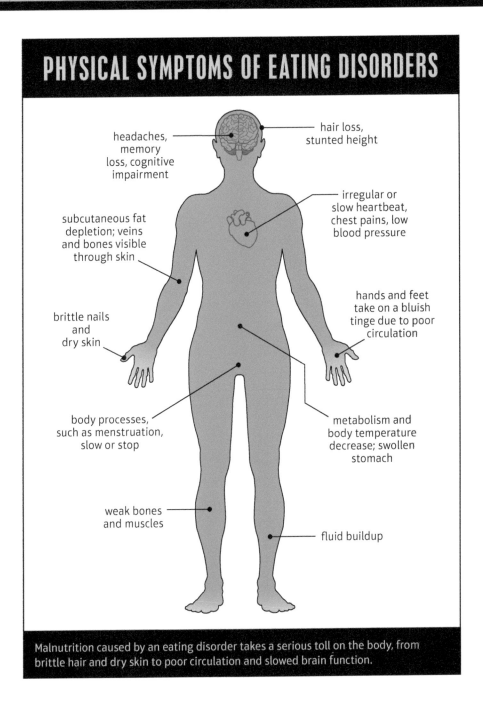

PHYSICAL SYMPTOMS OF EATING DISORDERS

headaches, memory loss, cognitive impairment

hair loss, stunted height

irregular or slow heartbeat, chest pains, low blood pressure

subcutaneous fat depletion; veins and bones visible through skin

hands and feet take on a bluish tinge due to poor circulation

brittle nails and dry skin

body processes, such as menstruation, slow or stop

metabolism and body temperature decrease; swollen stomach

weak bones and muscles

fluid buildup

Malnutrition caused by an eating disorder takes a serious toll on the body, from brittle hair and dry skin to poor circulation and slowed brain function.

The frontal lobe of the brain, which regulates impulse control, judgment, and organization, continues developing into a person's mid-twenties. Eating disorders can delay this development, which affects an individual's cognitive ability. People with eating disorders may show symptoms such as mental slowdown and distraction. The effects of an eating disorder on the brain can be permanent.

Effects Specific to Bulimia

Beyond the previously listed symptoms common with any eating disorder, bulimia comes with its own particular side effects. If someone repeatedly uses a finger to cause vomiting, the nails can scratch the throat and roof of the mouth. Repeated vomiting causes painful cracks in the corners of the mouth, called cheilosis.

Repeated vomiting can also damage the teeth and gums. Stomach acid in vomit wears down tooth enamel. The gums become inflamed. Many people with bulimia brush their teeth immediately after vomiting. This wears the enamel down even faster and can also make gums recede. Dentists can often easily spot someone who purges from tooth and gum damage. Some people even require caps on their teeth or oral surgery to repair their gums.

Repeated vomiting causes an enlargement of salivary glands. The parotid glands are in front of and below each ear. When they swell, the person's face looks distorted. Often even after someone has stopped purging, the glands remain permanently swollen.

Dr. Gerald Russell, responsible for first identifying bulimia, noted scarring on the tops of the hands of people who were repeatedly purging. The scars were caused by teeth rubbing on the hands repeatedly. These scars are called Russell's sign.

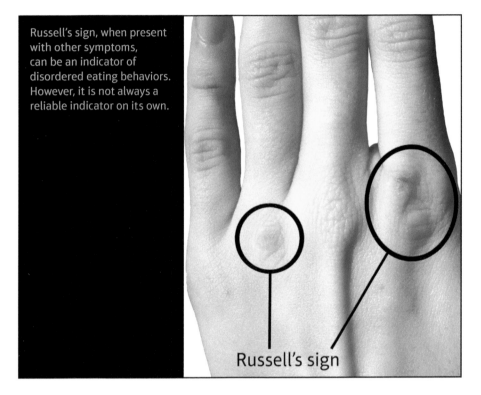

Russell's sign, when present with other symptoms, can be an indicator of disordered eating behaviors. However, it is not always a reliable indicator on its own.

Russell's sign

DAMAGE TO THE STOMACH AND ESOPHAGUS

The lower esophageal sphincter is a muscle that prevents stomach contents from flowing backward into the esophagus. When the sphincter is weakened by repeated vomiting, stomach acid can flow back into the esophagus. It causes a burning sensation in the chest called heartburn, or reflux. Some people develop sores, or ulcers, in the esophagus as a result of regular heartburn. This narrows the esophagus, making it harder to swallow food.

Repeated vomiting can also cause irritation or small tears in the esophagus and stomach. These can leave a person feeling weak, to the point where they may faint. They can also lead to anemia—an abnormally low level of red blood cells.

Tears in the esophagus and stomach are extremely serious because they can go undetected and can be deadly if left unaddressed. Smaller tears can cause internal bleeding. Eventually, a tear in the esophagus can burst. If this happens, stomach contents can surround the heart and lungs. A major tear in the stomach can cause the contents to flow into the abdominal cavity.

CULTURAL COMPETENCY

Historically, marginalized populations have been improperly treated for health conditions, due in part to biases reinforced in medical school and postgraduate training. Cultural differences between health care providers and patients can inadvertently result in lower-quality care. There is currently a movement in the medical field toward providing culturally competent health care. This type of care seeks to provide effective and quality health care to people of diverse backgrounds. It requires health care providers to understand how cultural differences may affect health outcomes. For example, a person's socioeconomic background, sexuality, or fluency in a language may influence how often they seek care, whom they feel comfortable sharing medical information with, and the likelihood that they will follow doctor recommendations.

The growing diversity of the US population means that health care providers need to be able to address a wide variety of patient needs. Cultural competence offers a framework so that patients can receive the best possible care for them as individuals.

Effects Specific to Binge Eating Disorder

People with binge eating disorder can experience numerous physical effects. They may be overweight or obese, but they may also be a healthy weight. If someone is experiencing binge eating disorder and is also overweight or obese, they may face health issues associated with carrying excess weight such as hypertension, elevated risk of heart disease, type 2 diabetes, and joint pain.

EMOTIONAL EFFECTS

The main effects of binge eating disorder are emotional and mental. Someone experiencing binge eating disorder may feel out of control around food; have feelings of anxiety, guilt, or depression related to their eating habits; or eat in secret. The psychological and psychosocial effects of binge eating disorder may result in social isolation, poor quality of life, and difficulties functioning at work or in their personal life.

CHAPTER SIX

TREATMENT

If an eating disorder is caught and treated early, there is a good chance of a fast and complete recovery. Unfortunately, this is not what usually happens. Eating disorders can go undiagnosed for a long time, sometimes for years. The biggest challenge in treating an eating disorder is for the person to recognize that their eating behaviors are problematic. Most people with an eating disorder deny that they need help. This can be especially true when they are neither under- nor overweight. They may have a misguided understanding of what constitutes an eating disorder. They may feel as though it's impossible for them to have an eating disorder if they are not below a certain weight. This is a myth and can lead to people causing irreparable damage to their bodies without realizing it. Eating disorders affect people of all shapes and sizes. The fact is people with eating disorders often do not enter treatment until a physical or mental crisis occurs.

EATING DISORDER HELPLINES

NEDA provides an eating disorder helpline at 800-931-2237. Volunteers are trained to provide support, resources, and treatment options for individuals or for those looking to help a loved one with an eating disorder. In addition to the phone line, the organization offers online chat and texting options.

The National Suicide Prevention Lifeline is a toll-free hotline in the United States for people who are in distress and at risk of harming themselves. The service has a network of over 160 crisis centers across the country. Anyone can call the lifeline by dialing 988 and connect with a trained crisis worker at their nearest crisis center. Conversations are confidential, and workers are trained to be active, nonjudgmental listeners. They can also provide resources to callers concerned about a friend or family member.

For those who prefer to communicate by text, the Crisis Text Line is a free and confidential service where trained crisis counselors provide support. The text line is available through Facebook Messenger, WhatsApp, and text message at 741741.

These resources are intended to provide people with support in cases where immediate medical attention is not needed. If you or someone you know is experiencing a medical emergency or has a plan for suicide, call 911 immediately.

Eating disorders come with a complicated mix of physical and psychological symptoms. An underlying psychological disorder can make it difficult to untangle a pattern of disordered eating, and the physical effects of an eating disorder can cause changes to a person's attitudes and emotions. For this reason, eating disorder treatment addresses both the mind and body.

Finding a doctor who specializes in treating eating disorders is important. A family doctor or pediatrician without training in eating disorders may not be aware of all the available treatment options. Recovery is a team effort. In the best scenario a team of doctors works together to treat someone with an eating disorder. The eating disorder specialist leads the team, coordinating with doctors to provide a treatment plan that addresses the behavioral,

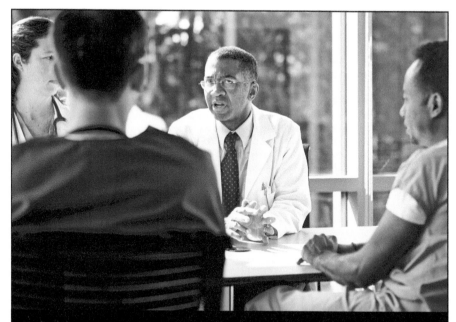

Medical doctors, psychologists, and nutritionists often work in coordination when determining a treatment plan for a patient with an eating disorder.

psychological, physical, and social aspects of the eating disorder. A therapist provides counseling for patients and their families. A nutritionist monitors meal planning and overall nutrition. Some therapists and nutritionists specialize in treating people with eating disorders.

Treatment Approaches

Once doctors have diagnosed a patient with an eating disorder, the patient and caregivers choose a treatment approach. Each patient is different, and no one treatment plan works for all cases. A patient's recovery team should investigate all available methods and customize the treatment for the patient. A person with an eating disorder may have a hard time making important decisions alone. If there is a good family environment, it can be helpful to involve the family in treatment decisions as well.

First, the team must deal with physical symptoms and restore proper nutrition. Ensuring the patient is on the way to a healthy diet and out of physical danger is the first goal. Then therapy can begin, either individually, with a group, or with family.

Where treatment takes place depends on the severity of the disorder. When an eating disorder is diagnosed early, patients can remain at home. They attend sessions at a therapist's office for several hours each week. Some patients live at home but attend sessions at a clinic for most of the day. They eat most meals at the clinic. When physical symptoms are more serious, patients may need to be treated at the hospital for several hours each day. In the most serious cases, patients are treated at a facility that specializes in eating disorders. They live in the hospital full-time until they have made enough improvement, both physically and mentally, to go home. Patients might stay at these facilities for long periods, from a few weeks to several months.

Medical Treatment

There is no single medication that can cure an eating disorder. Medication can be part of a treatment plan that combines therapy and nutritional counseling. But doctors need to be careful when prescribing medications. Malnutrition changes how medicines affect the mind and body. It also affects mood and behavior. This can make it difficult to determine if a patient has any underlying emotional issues that doctors would treat with medication.

Doctors sometimes prescribe antidepressants to treat eating disorders. They help increase the level of serotonin in the brain and have been proven to help treat bulimia. Antidepressants are often used in conjunction with other treatments to help alleviate symptoms of depression or anxiety that may be present in someone experiencing an eating disorder.

HOSPITALIZATION AND REFEEDING

It may take a life-threatening incident for a person with an eating disorder to accept the help they need. Someone dealing with a restrictive eating disorder may experience chest pains, fainting, have a heart attack, or attempt suicide. For someone with bulimia, a tear in the esophagus, the stomach, or vomiting blood can be fatal. Hospitalization provides the patient with protection and treatment.

Once someone with an eating disorder is admitted to a hospital, doctors will begin reintroducing the patient to normal eating behaviors. This is called refeeding. The toll an eating disorder takes on the body is considerable—lost nutrients; internal damage from purging; and muscle, tissue, and organ reduction. This damage must be repaired before other forms of recovery can begin. Repairing internal damage takes time and patience.

A nutritionist works with the patient to plan a menu, often a combination of liquid food supplements and solid foods. The nutritionist will try to accommodate the person with "safe foods," or foods that the person enjoys or feels comfortable eating.

Refeeding can be traumatic for the patient. They may not want to eat. They may be very angry that they are in the hospital and may insist that nothing is wrong. Eating attempts may make them anxious and fearful. Someone with anorexia has generally been eating very little. The thought of eating a normal diet, which could be several times the number of calories they had been consuming, may be terrifying. Refeeding must be done slowly and carefully. The body has adapted to starvation. A rapid increase in consumption can worsen electrolyte and other biochemical balances and can cause abdominal pain and bloating. Doctors recommend a slow refeeding process for an average weight gain of about 2 to 3 pounds (0.9 to 1.4 kg) a week.

Psychotherapy

Psychotherapy is a critical part of treatment. It provides a safe environment for talking about any topic without fear of consequences. During traditional psychotherapy, a psychologist examines a patient's subconscious mind to discover the roots of a psychological problem. The therapist might interpret dreams and analyze hidden feelings. This type of therapy focuses on past traumas or unresolved issues from childhood or adolescence that might have contributed to the eating disorder. One of the goals of

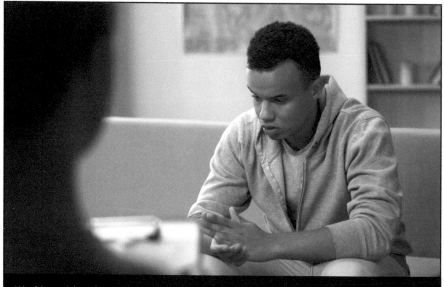

Working with a therapist can help a patient address emotional and psychological challenges that may be contributing to disordered eating behaviors.

psychotherapy is to identify and resolve the issues that triggered the eating disorder.

Low self-esteem is often identified as a major issue for people with eating disorders. Psychotherapy can address the root causes of low self-esteem to improve a patient's mental well-being. It can also help to identify other psychological disorders that may have contributed to the eating disorder. Depression, obsessive-compulsive disorder, and anxiety often go hand in hand with eating disorders. A therapist can help sort out which emotional and mood problems were caused by the eating disorder and which existed prior to it. There is no one-size-fits-all approach to treating an eating disorder. Each individual situation must be evaluated by the treatment team to determine which type of therapy might be most effective.

COGNITIVE BEHAVIORAL THERAPY

Cognitive behavioral therapy (CBT) is one of the most widely used therapies in treating eating disorders. It can also be used to treat co-occurring disorders, such as depression, OCD, and anxiety. CBT is based on the idea that thoughts (cognition) and actions (behaviors) are related. When we change our thoughts around a certain subject, we can also change our behaviors. Once the relationships between thoughts, emotions, and actions are understood, the patient can replace negative thoughts and emotions with positive ones. The patient can begin to return to a healthy lifestyle.

CBT teaches patients that environmental factors such as family and school are not responsible for their thoughts or behavior. Instead, CBT teaches individuals that they alone are responsible for their own recovery. This approach can be comforting and empowering to individuals who feel that their lives are out of their control. With CBT, individuals learn which situations can trigger stress, how to avoid those situations as much as possible, and how to tolerate them when they are unavoidable. Using these techniques helps patients to avoid a relapse into disordered eating.

The Maudsley Family-Based Approach

The Maudsley family-based approach is named for the London hospital where it was developed in the 1980s. It is specifically for children or teenagers living at home.

The Maudsley approach is grounded in the idea that the eating disorder controls the patient, rather than the other way around. The patient did not choose to stop eating and is not able to change their behavior. To that end, parents must take control from the eating disorder so that it becomes powerless. In the early stages of treatment, parents are responsible for dispensing all food, and the child must be monitored full-time for the first few weeks. Gradually, as the patient gains weight, they also regain control over their individual eating habits. Once they are able to maintain a healthy weight, treatment begins to focus more on helping the patient develop a positive and healthy identity.

Other Treatments

Patients often undergo other types of treatment along with those already mentioned. Other treatments include physical or occupational therapy, art therapy, yoga, and meditation. Twelve-step programs, life coaches, and biofeedback are other alternatives.

A twelve-step program is a specific course of action for recovery from substance use or behavior problems. The founders of Alcoholics Anonymous created the twelve-step program, but people recovering from other addictions use the program as well. For people with eating disorders, the steps can help them to identify the problem, accept that they need help, examine past behaviors, and work to find an emotional and behavioral process that reduces the chance of relapse.

Life coaches are trained to help people achieve personal and emotional goals. Coaching typically addresses attitude-related thoughts and behaviors that act as barriers to reaching those goals, such as negative beliefs and self-talk. An individual may choose to use a life coach to establish personal accountability and inspire positive change in their life.

Biofeedback is a technique that uses special instruments to measure a person's heart rate, brain activity, muscle tension,

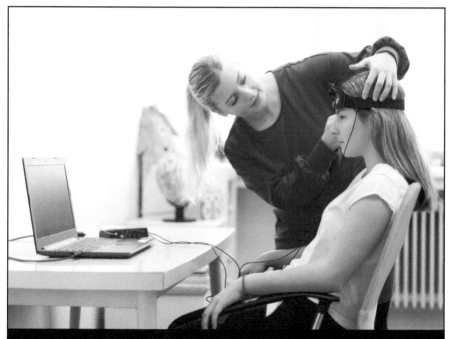

During a biofeedback session, a therapist uses electronic sensors to monitor bodily functions. They may use interactive computer programs to help patients develop stress reduction techniques.

and skin temperature. It provides information on how a person's body reacts to physical or psychological stress. The idea is that once people are aware of how they physically feel when they are stressed, they can make physical changes to reduce that stress. For example, if a person knows that they tend to take shallow breaths and tense their shoulders when stressed, they may focus on relaxing their shoulders and taking longer, deeper breaths when they encounter stressful situations.

CONCLUSION

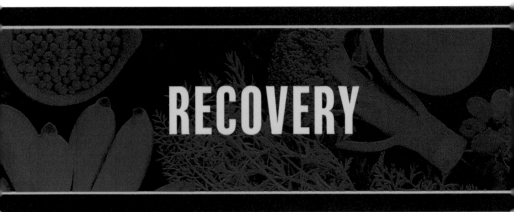

RECOVERY

Recovering from an eating disorder is difficult and takes time and patience. It involves more than an end to disordered eating behaviors such as bingeing, purging, and food restriction. It means addressing unhealthy attitudes around food and weight as well.

Trying to eliminate longtime behaviors and beliefs takes courage, perseverance, and the support of family and friends. There is no "normal" recovery time from any eating disorder. Recovery is quicker for some people than others. For many people, recovering from an eating disorder is challenging and can take significant time.

Relapse

Most people being treated for an eating disorder have at least one relapse. It is important to recognize that recovery from an eating disorder is often not linear. After an eating disorder is recognized, acknowledged, and diagnosed, a person may go through several cycles of recovery and relapse. The number of times a person falls back into unhealthy eating patterns and negative thoughts is not important. A good therapist will assure their patients that recovery is a gradual process with ups and downs. Relapsing does not mean failure. Instead, they can use the relapse as an opportunity to identify and eliminate the triggers for abnormal eating behaviors.

Symptoms of relapse include weight loss, disordered eating behaviors, and distorted attitudes regarding body weight and shape. Someone may develop symptoms of a different eating disorder during their relapse. One common issue for people being treated for an eating disorder is overexercising. A person in recovery might take up exercise as a healthy way to take care of their bodies. However, this can become a replacement for restriction or purging.

The best way to minimize or prevent relapse is to identify risky situations in advance. Risky situations are usually something external. They can range from a big event—a breakup, for example— to something like the tone of someone's voice. If the person in recovery knows that particular situations or interactions have caused stress or triggered disordered eating behaviors in the past, they can take steps to avoid or better manage those situations and interactions in the future.

Chronic Health Issues

Some people, depending on the type, length, and physical symptoms of their eating disorder, may experience long-term health problems. These can include issues related to infertility, bone

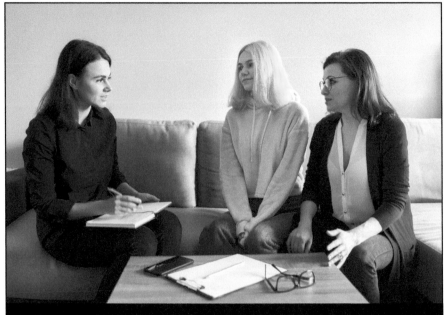

Establishing and maintaining a long-term support system can help reduce the likelihood of relapse into disordered eating behaviors. This support system may include a regularly visited therapist, family members, friends, or support groups.

density, weakened heart muscle, damage to the digestive tract, and other organ damage.

Some people who have recovered from an eating disorder still experience depression, anxiety, or compulsive behavior. Many times these issues contributed to developing the eating disorder in the first place. Focusing on food restriction or bingeing and purging helped the person avoid these issues. Stopping the disordered eating does not mean the underlying issues are gone. Once the disordered eating behavior is treated, a person can address underlying issues openly and in a healthy way. Anyone going through recovery with a therapist will work to understand and manage these other mental health issues.

Supporting Recovery

It may be difficult for someone going through recovery to reenter their life and try to navigate through the constant messaging from society—and maybe even their friends and family—that normalizes disordered eating patterns or promoting thinness as an ideal of beauty or health. It may be helpful for them to speak out about their experience. Sharing their story with family and friends can help destigmatize eating disorders and may also help communities start to combat societal ideas of what is healthy, normal, or beautiful. Others may find meaning in being able to offer their support and understanding to people who are currently recovering from their own eating disorders.

Anyone who does not have an eating disorder but would like to work toward a healthier society in general can help by challenging views on health, healthy or normal eating patterns, and ideas of what a normal weight or normal body might look like. They might also take the time to educate themselves about eating disorders, culture that promotes disordered eating, body positivity and body neutrality movements, anti-fatphobia and fat liberation movements, and other movements that seek to reevaluate societal and medical standards.

Each person who is experiencing or has experienced an eating disorder will have their own challenges on the road to recovery. Some people may battle thoughts and behaviors related to their eating disorder, as well as triggers, for their entire lives. The goal of treatment is always for the individual to lead a life free of eating disorder thoughts and behaviors. Recovery takes time and patience, but it is possible, and the rewards are well worth it.

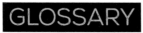

GLOSSARY

anorexia nervosa: a life-threatening eating disorder characterized by self-starvation and excessive weight loss

bingeing: consuming an atypically large quantity of food in a short period of time; eating uncontrollably

biofeedback: a technique in which people learn to control certain internal bodily processes that normally occur involuntarily, such as heart rate, blood pressure, muscle tension, and skin temperature

bipolar disorder: a disorder wherein people experience extreme moods, swinging between depression and mania

bulimia: repeated overeating binges followed by compensatory behavior, such as forced vomiting or excessive exercise

cortisol: a hormone that regulates stress and anxiety

dehydration: the loss of water and salts from the body

depression: a mood disorder that is usually expressed by feelings of worthlessness, sadness, irritability, inappropriate guilt, lack of motivation, and disturbed sleep

diuretics: medication that works to remove fluid from the body through urination

eating disorder: extreme emotions, attitudes, and behavior surrounding eating, food, and weight

electrolytes: minerals that conduct electricity and are found in various fluids and tissues throughout the body

emaciated: thin and feeble, especially due to illness

esophagus: a hollow, muscular tube that starts in the throat and ends at the stomach

fasting: abstaining from food

genetics: the study of heredity, the process in which biological parents pass certain genes on to their children

glucose: a type of sugar used for energy and found in the blood

hormones: chemicals released by cells that affect cells in other parts in the body

hysteria: a medical term that is used to refer to a state of extreme fear or emotion and irrational behavior

lanugo: a fine, downy body hair

leptin: a hormone that regulates appetite and weight

malnutrition: when the body does not get enough nutrients

metabolism: all the physical and chemical processes in the body that create and use energy

neurotransmitter: a chemical in the brain used as a messenger from one nerve cell to another

obsessive-compulsive disorder (OCD): a disorder wherein obsessions (recurrent and intrusive thoughts, feelings, ideas, or actions) constantly occupy the mind of the individual

osteoporosis: a disease in which the density and quality of bone are reduced

purging: self-induced vomiting or defecating

refeeding: restarting nutrition to someone with an eating disorder

relapse: when someone who is getting treatment for a problem slips back into the disordered behavior or thinking

restriction: limiting food to an extreme degree

serotonin: a hormone in the brain that communicates between nerve cells; a neurotransmitter

twelve-step program: a set of guiding principles outlining a course of action for recovery from substance use, compulsion, or other behavioral problems

SOURCE NOTES

12 Tom Wooldridge, "Anorexia Nervosa: Not Just for Women!" *Psychology Today*, October 14, 2012, https://www.psychologytoday.com/us/blog /the-forgotten-gender/201210/anorexia-nervosa-not-just-women.

17 Gerald Russell, "Bulimia Nervosa: An Ominous Variant of Anorexia Nervosa," *Psychological Medicine* 9, no. 3 (August 1979): 429–448, https://pubmed.ncbi.nlm.nih.gov/482466/.

25 Angela Guarda, "Expert Q & A: Eating Disorders," American Psychiatric Association, December 2020, https://www.psychiatry .org/patients-families/eating-disorders/expert-q-and-a.

34 April Fulton, "When Efforts to Eat 'Clean' Become an Unhealthy Obsession," NPR, October 7, 2019, https://www.npr.org/sections /thesalt/2019/10/07/766847274/when-efforts-to-eat-clean -become-an-unhealthy-obsession.

39 Jamie Reno, "Eating Disorders Among Teens Have Risen During COVID-19: What Parents Can Do," Healthline, May 16, 2021, https://www.healthline.com/health-news/eating-disorders -among-teens-have-risen-during-covid-19-what-parents-can-do.

39 Jamie Reno, "Eating Disorders Among Teens Have Risen During COVID-19: What Parents Can Do," Healthline, May 16, 2021, https://www.healthline.com/health-news/eating-disorders -among-teens-have-risen-during-covid-19-what-parents-can-do.

51 Alex Rodriguez, "Sorry and Deeply Regretful," interview by Peter Gammons, *SportsCenter*, ESPN, February 9, 2009, https://www .espn.com/mlb/news/story?id=3895281.

52 Sarah Marsh, "Eating Disorders in Men Rise by 70% in NHS Figures," *The Guardian*, July 31, 2017, https://www.theguardian .com/society/2017/jul/31/eating-disorders-in-men-rise-by-70 -in-nhs-figures.

56   Cathy Rigby McCoy, "A Onetime Olympic Gymnast Overcomes
     the Bulimia that Threatened Her Life," *People*, August 13, 1984,
     https://people.com/archive/a-onetime-olympic-gymnas
     t-overcomes-the-bulimia-that-threatened-her-life-vol-22-no-7/.

60   "Not All Black Girls Know How to Eat," *Student Life* (blog), National
     Eating Disorders Association, accessed February 14, 2022,
     https://www.nationaleatingdisorders.org/blog/not-all-black-girls
     -know-how-eat.

RESOURCES

Eating Disorder Hope
https://www.eatingdisorderhope.com
This informative website is dedicated to educating and spreading awareness about eating disorders and helping those with eating disorders to navigate their personal eating disorder recovery.

National Eating Disorder Information Centre
https://nedic.ca
This Canadian site provides help, support, and information on eating disorders.

National Eating Disorders Association
http://www.nationaleatingdisorders.org
The National Eating Disorders Association provides information and resources on eating disorders, including a kit for parents and other family members, links to treatment centers, referrals to health professionals where you live, and much more.

National Institute of Mental Health, "Eating Disorders"
https://www.nimh.nih.gov/health/topics/eating-disorders
This website provides expert information and resources about bulimia, anorexia nervosa, and binge eating disorder.

Something Fishy: Website on Eating Disorders
http://www.something-fishy.org
This comprehensive site is dedicated to providing awareness and support to people with eating disorders.

SELECTED BIBLIOGRAPHY

ABC News. "Young Girls Start Eating Disorders Early." ABC, January 6, 2006. https://abcnews.go.com/GMA/story?id=126486&page=1.

Bennett, Jessica. "Debunking the Myths of Anorexia." *Newsweek*, September 5, 2008. https://www.newsweek.com/debunking-myths-anorexia-88909.

Boskind-White, Marlene, and William C. White Jr. *Bulimia/Anorexia: The Binge-Purge Cycle and Self-Starvation*. 5th ed. New York: W. W. Norton, 2001.

"Eating Disorder Statistics." National Association of Anorexia Nervosa and Associated Disorders. Accessed December 13, 2021. https://anad.org /education-and-awareness/about-eating-disorders/eating-disorders -statistics/.

Fuller, Kristen. "We Are Failing at Treating Eating Disorders in Minorities." *Psychology Today*, February 28, 2019. https://www.psychologytoday.com /us/blog/happiness-is-state-mind/201902/we-are-failing-treating-eating -disorders-in-minorities.

Guarda, Angela, physician reviewer. "What Are Eating Disorders?" American Psychiatric Association. March 2021. https://www.psychiatry.org/patients -families/eating-disorders/what-are-eating-disorders.

Harding, Anne. "Eating Disorder May Be Missed in Boys, Non-whites." *Reuters Health*, May 11, 2007. https://www.reuters.com/article/us-eating-disorder -boys-non-whites-idUSARM16962320070511.

Heaton, Jeanne A., and Claudia J. Strauss. *Talking to Eating Disorders: Simple Ways to Support Someone with Anorexia, Bulimia, Binge Eating, or Body Image Issues*. New York: New American Library, 2005.

Jargon, Julie. "Boys Have Eating Disorders, Too. Doctors Think Social Media Is Making It Worse." *Wall Street Journal*, November 13, 2021. https://www.wsj .com/articles/boys-have-eating-disorders-too-doctors-think-social-media -is-making-it-worse-11636812000.

Jones, Clay. "A British Teenager is Blind, but Not Because of Junk Food or 'Fussy Eating.'" Science-Based Medicine. September 6, 2019. https://sciencebasedmedicine.org/a-british-teenager-is-blind-but-not-because-of-junk-food-or-fussy-eating.

Mayo Clinic. "Anorexia Nervosa." Accessed December 13, 2021. https://www.mayoclinic.org/diseases-conditions/anorexia-nervosa/symptoms-causes/syc-20353591.

National Eating Disorders Association. "Health Consequences." Accessed January 28, 2022. https://www.nationaleatingdisorders.org/health-consequences.

National Eating Disorders Association. "Identity and Eating Disorders." Accessed December 13, 2021. https://www.nationaleatingdisorders.org/identity-eating-disorders.

National Eating Disorders Association. "Statistics and Research on Eating Disorders." Accessed December 13, 2021. https://www.nationaleatingdisorders.org/statistics-research-eating-disorders.

National Eating Disorders Association. "Warning Signs and Symptoms." Accessed December 13, 2021. https://www.nationaleatingdisorders.org/warning-signs-and-symptoms.

Scaccia, Annamarya. "What Are Pro-Ana Sites and Why Are They So Dangerous?" Healthline. February 21, 2018. https://www.healthline.com/health/why-pro-ana-sites-are-so-dangerous.

University of Virginia. "Adolescent Girls with ADHD Are at Increased Risk for Eating Disorders, Study Shows." ScienceDaily. March 15, 2008. http://www.sciencedaily.com/releases/2008/03/080314085032.htm.

FURTHER READING

Books for Young Adults

Bacon, Lindo. *Health at Every Size: The Surprising Truth about Your Weight.* Dallas: BenBella Books, 2010.

Edut, Ophira, ed. *Body Outlaws: Rewriting the Rules of Beauty and Body Image.* Emeryville, CA: Seal Press, 2003.

Gaudiani, Jennifer L. *Sick Enough: A Guide to the Medical Complications of Eating Disorders.* New York: Routledge, 2019.

Gay, Roxane. *Hunger: A Memoir of (My) Body.* New York: Harper, 2017.

Gordon, Aubrey. *What We Don't Talk about When We Talk about Fat.* Boston: Beacon Press, 2020.

Tandoh, Ruby. *Eat Up! Food, Appetite, and Eating What You Want.* London: Serpent's Tail, 2018.

Tovar, Virgie. *You Have the Right to Remain Fat.* New York: Feminist Press, 2018.

Books for Parents and Family Members

Bell, Lara Lyn. *By Their Side: A Resource for Caretakers and Loved Ones Facing an Eating Disorder.* Dallas: Brown Books Publishing Group, 2019.

Shavin, Dana Lise. *The Body Tourist.* New York: Little Feather Books, 2014.

Siegel, Michele Judith Brisman, and Margot Weinshel. *Surviving an Eating Disorder: Strategies for Family and Friends.* New York: Collins Living, 2009.

Strings, Sabrina. *Fearing the Black Body: The Racial Origins of Fat Phobia.* New York: New York University Press, 2019.

Websites

Centre for Clinical Interventions, "Disordered Eating"
https://www.cci.health.wa.gov.au/Resources/Looking-After-Yourself/Disordered-Eating
This resource page is hosted by the Government of Western Australia. It includes online modules for navigating eating disorders. The modules explain disordered eating behaviors and outline methods for challenging unhealthy behaviors and mindsets.

Eating Disorder Therapy LA, "Recommended Reading and Resources"
https://www.eatingdisordertherapyla.com/reading-resources
The resources listed at this website are meant to supplement therapy
treatment for eating disorders. Readers can learn more about cognitive
behavioral therapy, the Maudsley method, medical complications caused
by eating disorders, and more. Digital resources such as podcasts and
recovery apps are also listed.

Eating Disorders Resource Catalogue
https://www.edcatalogue.com
The Eating Disorders Resource Catalogue is home to hundreds of
inspirational and informational articles about eating disorder recovery.
Articles are written by leading experts in the field as well as recovered
and recovering individuals willing to share their personal experiences.
The site also provides the names and addresses of eating disorder
organizations and treatment facilities.

Eating Disorders Resource Center (EDRC)
https://edrcsv.org
EDRC is a non-profit organization that provides resources, information,
and support for those experiencing eating disorders. They facilitate
support groups for those in recovery as well as education and outreach
programs.

The Lily, "Fat People Have Eating Disorders, Too. Why Don't We Talk about
Them?"
https://www.thelily.com/fat-people-have-eating-disorders-too-why-dont
-we-talk-about-them
This article, written by Amanda Scriver, analyzes the ways that society's
misconceptions about weight and disordered eating cause eating
disorders to be overlooked in plus-sized women.

National Eating Disorders Association (NEDA)
https://www.nationaleatingdisorders.org
NEDA seeks to raise awareness about eating disorders by providing
programs and services for individuals with eating disorders and their
families. They also fund research and advocate for additional education
related to eating disorders in schools. Readers can find out more data
about eating disorders and learn how to get involved in awareness efforts.

National Suicide Prevention Lifeline
https://suicidepreventionlifeline.org
This site has information about suicide and a search tool for finding a crisis center near you. There is also a toll-free, twenty-four-hour hotline for those in crisis or thinking about suicide.

Nutrition Journal, "Weight Science: Evaluating the Evidence for a Paradigm Shift"
https://nutritionj.biomedcentral.com/articles/10.1186/1475-2891-10-9
This 2011 study, which appeared in the peer-reviewed academic journal *Nutrition Journal*, found that medical guidelines that focus on weight and weight loss are not only ineffective at producing healthier, thinner bodies, but may also contribute to harmful outcomes such as low self-esteem and disordered eating. The article suggests that alternative, weight-neutral guidelines may lead to better health outcomes.

Psychology Today, "Find a Therapist"
https://www.psychologytoday.com/us/therapists
This site helps connect patients with therapists in the United States. The website allows users to filter potential therapists by location, specialty, health insurance coverage, and more.

Scientific American, "In Obesity Research, Fatphobia Is Always the X Factor"
https://www.scientificamerican.com/article/in-obesity-research
-fatphobia-is-always-the-x-factor/
This *Scientific American* article delves into how stigma around weight can impact the design—and therefore results—of medical research studies.

INDEX

ABOUT THE AUTHORS

Carol Sonenklar's first young adult books were inspired by her two children. She has since written about a wide range of subjects including health, the environment, and popular history. She enjoys translating complex topics into understandable and engaging writing. Sonenklar is also an editor and specializes in helping writers for whom English is a second language. Sonenklar loves to hike with her two dogs in the mountains. She currently lives in Colorado.

Tabitha Moriarty is a medical student living in Atlanta, Georgia.

PHOTO ACKNOWLEDGMENTS

Image credits: Muslim Girl/Getty Images, p. 5; DiferentRoger/Shutterstock.com, p. 7; duncan1890/Getty Images, p. 13; Denver Post/Getty Images, p. 16; Harry Langdon/Getty Images, p. 19; H.S. Photos/Alamy Stock Photo, p. 21; pickingpok/Shutterstock.com, p. 25; DGLimages/Getty Images, p. 26; Martin Novak/Getty Images, p. 29; dmphoto/Getty Images, p. 33; BSIP/Getty Images, p. 37; Enrico Calderoni/Getty Images, p. 41; Gonzalo Marroquin/Getty Images, p. 45; Mariia Boiko/Alamy Stock Photo, p. 46; SolStock/Getty Images, p. 49; Focus On Sport/Getty Images, p. 51; Fran Polito/Getty Images, p. 54; Bettmann/Getty Images, p. 56; Federico Rotter/NurPhoto/Getty Images, p. 61; Motortion Films/Shutterstock.com, p. 62; Ralf Liebhold/Shutterstock.com, p. 69; Wikimedia Commons/Kyukyusha, p. 73; Thomas Barwick/Getty Images, p. 78; Andrea Obzerova/500px/Getty Images, p. 85; Valeriy_G/iStock/Getty Images, p. 88. Cover images: Lesterman/Shutterstock.com; Marco Brockmann/Shutterstock.com.